Statistics in Medical Research

Developments in Clinical Trials

Statistics in Medical Research

Developments in Clinical Trials

Edmund A. Gehan, Ph.D., *and*
Noreen A. Lemak, M.D.

The University of Texas
M.D. Anderson Cancer Center
Houston, Texas

Plenum Medical Book Company • New York and London

Library of Congress Cataloging-in-Publication Data

Statistics in medical research : developments in clinical trials /
 Edmund A. Gehan and Noreen A. Lemak.
      p.   cm.
   Includes bibliographical references and index.
   ISBN 0-306-44863-7
   1. Medicine--Statistical methods--History. 2. Clinical trials-
 -Statistical methods--History.   I. Gehan, Edmund A. II. Lemak,
 Noreen A.
 R853.S7S777   1994
 610'.72--dc20   94-40009
                                                            CIP

To my wife, Brenda;
and my children,
James, Laura, Carole, Diane, and Margery
—EAG

To my husband, Leslie;
and my children,
Michael, Margaret, and Robert
— NAL

ISBN 0-306-44863-7

© 1994 Plenum Publishing Corporation
233 Spring Street, New York, N. Y. 10013

Plenum Medical Book Company is an imprint of Plenum Publishing Corporation

Printed in the United States of America

Preface

In 1890, General Francis A. Walker, president of both the Massachusetts Institute of Technology and the American Statistical Association, wrote

> There is reason to wish that all citizens, from the highest to the lowest, might undergo so much of training in statistics as should enable them to detect the errors lurking in quantitative statements regarding social and economic matters which may . . . be addressed to them as voters or as critics of public policies. [F. A. Walker, 1890; reprinted in Noether, 1989]

It has been more than a century since Walker stated his wish, but progress has been slow, just as advancement in the establishment of statistical principles and methodology has been laborious and difficult over the centuries.

We have tried to describe the milestones in this development and how each generation of scientists built on the heritage and foundations laid by their predecessors. Many historians dismiss the "great man theory," which alleges that giant "leaps of human knowledge are made by great thinkers who transcend the boundaries of their times; great scientists don't leap outside their time, but somewhere else in their own time" (Hevly, 1990). We found this to be the case in the history of statistics. Even the innovative writings of Karl Pearson and Sir Ronald Fisher that became the foundation of modern mathematical statistics were the outcome of two centuries of antecedent ideas and information.

We were interested in discovering how an idea was introduced and how it then spread and generated new conceptions among men of varied cultures whose backgrounds and education had prepared them to grasp the idea and advance it. When controversies occurred (as in the section in Chapter 5 on randomized versus historical controls in clinical trials), we have tried to present both sides.

Some scientists described in our book had doubts about the value of statistics. Could statistics even be considered a science? When the Statistical Society of London was founded in 1834, the members decided that as long as statisticians limited their sphere to the acquisition, cataloging, and presentation of data, that was science. If statisticians began interpreting findings, that would be "argumentation, with passions and politics entering, and that was not science" (Cochran, 1982). As recently as 1924, Major Greenwood asked, "Is the scientific method of value in medical research?" (Greenwood, 1924).

Writing a historical book is truly a labor of love. The background research is entertaining and enjoyable because medical articles from the past include long, vivid descriptions of patients or diseases, and the narratives have much ornamenting, often anecdotal, that sometimes carries the reader into philosophy, ethics, or other areas far afield from the stated topic. But you learn a lot and remember it easily. In contrast, the concise, state-the-facts-only approach used in medical journals today can often lead to very dull reading.

If a medical student reads Dr. John Locke's account of his nighttime house call to the Paris home of the English ambassador in 1677, the student will never forget the picture of an excruciating attack of trigeminal neuralgia; the violent and exquisite torment will be indelibly fixed in his or her memory. Similarly, in this book, we hope that our description of the introduction of modern statistics with the 1662 publication of John Graunt's *Natural and Political Observations on the London Bills of Mortality* (Chapter 1) will be remembered. Graunt described women who quarantined the diseased and investigated and reported deaths for the weekly Bills as "ancient matrons" whose diagnostic powers were affected by the "mist of a cup of Ale and the bribe of a two-groat fee."

Statistics has been shaped by many factors since its birth around the gambling tables, and various cultures and world events (e.g., epidemics, wars) influenced it. This book traces the historical development of statistics in medical research, but it is light reading, and we hope that you will enjoy it.

Edmund A. Gehan
Noreen A. Lemak

Acknowledgments

We are indebted to Emil J Freireich, M.D., for his encouragement and support and to Joan Fisher Box for her letters that included material used in Chapter 3 on her father, Sir Ronald Aylmer Fisher.

Also, we would like to thank Kimberly J. T. Herrick, Department of Scientific Publications at The University of Texas M. D. Anderson Cancer Center, for her valuable help.

This endeavor was supported in part by the National Institutes of Health Grants CA 30138 and CA 16672 and by the Kathryn O'Connor Research Fund.

Contents

CHAPTER 1

The Dawning of Statistics

The techniques and study designs used by statisticians today were gradually developed by scientists of vision over many centuries. Those pioneers understood and recorded many of the basic concepts of modern analytic logic. Often, ideas could not be tested or verified because the scientific world and society in general were not ready to accept them. As recently as the late 1940s, Sir Austin Bradford Hill "deliberately left out the words 'randomization' and 'random sampling numbers'" in his articles because he was "trying to persuade the doctors to come into controlled trials in the very simplest form and might have scared them off" (Hill, 1990).

> Despite the fact that some of the original data-collection systems pertained to information of interest to clinicians, clinical scientists were slow to embrace this new discipline [statistics]. Indeed, social scientists, agronomists, and astronomers were among the first to recognize the inherent variability in their data and to see the value of a systematic approach to analyzing and reporting such data. Consequently, statistical vocabulary is replete with terms whose origins make sense only when viewed from a historical perspective. [O'Fallon, 1988]

In this chapter we will review broadly the predecessor of our present-day clinical trials—the experiment performed on patients—using various therapies in an attempt to determine the relative merits of each. Perceptive students of earlier times were able to assess their observations and use sound reasoning to interpret them. Although they often arrived at correct diagnoses, their evaluations of treatments were limited by worthless remedies. It was not an inability to recognize a disease; they simply did not often have effective therapy (Crombie, 1961). Alongside our current imposing array of pharmaceuticals and surgical procedures, their drugs were relatively powerless, and surgery was limited by the lack of anesthesia and antisepsis.

Experience was the Judge

Aurelius Celsus (circa A.D. 25)

In *De Medicina*, one of the first medical books to be printed (1478), Celsus described therapeutics in his day—the first century A.D.—in the following way: "careful men noted what generally answered the better, and then began to prescribe the same for their patients" (Bull, 1959).

Avicenna (980–1037)

Avicenna, an Arabic scholar and author of an important medical work, *Canon*, described 760 drugs (Mettler, 1947), which were primarily herbs or dried animal tissues. He also presented some guidelines for drug trials, writing that a remedy should be used in its natural state on uncomplicated disease, that two opposed cases be observed, and that study be made of the time of action and of the reproducibility of the effects. He further stated, "The experimentation must be done with the human body, for testing a drug on a lion or a horse might not prove anything about its effect on man" (Crombie, 1952).

Philippus Aureolus Paracelsus (1493–1541)

Paracelsus recorded a belief similar to that of Celsus: "experience is the judge; if a thing stands the test of experience, it should be accepted; if it does not stand this test, it should be rejected" (Paracelsus, date unknown; Bull, 1959).

Ambroïse Paré (1510–1590)

Ambroïse Paré wrote one of the earliest reports of a clinical experiment, which occurred by chance.

> I had read that gunshot wounds were poisoned by the gunpowder and to cure them it was imperative to cauterize them with scalding

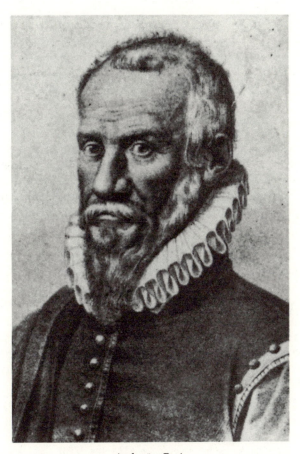

Ambroïse Paré.

hot oil of elders to which a little theriac had been added. . . . There came a time, however, that because I was without oil that I applied a dressing made of yolk of egg, oil of roses and turpentine. That night I could not sleep for I was troubled about the dressing and feared that the next morning I would find the patients dead, or close to death from the poison of the wound. I rose early, visited my patients and found those dressed with the "digestive" free of pain with uninflamed wounds—moreover they had rested all night. The patients treated with the scalding oil were feverish, in great pain and the area about their wound was swollen and inflamed. After I tried this many times I felt that neither I nor any other should ever cauterize gunshot wounds. [Malgaigne, 1840; Mettler, 1947, p. 845]

Francis Bacon, First Baron (1561–1626)

Francis Bacon wrote that both the time of germination and the vigor of the growth of wheat seeds were influenced by steeping them in different preparations (water mixed with cow dung, urine, and three dissimilar wines) with unsteeped seeds as controls. All wines were inferior; the winner was urine (Bacon, 1627; Cochran, 1976).

John Hunter (1728–1793)

John Hunter, who dominated surgery during the 1700s, described five cases in which he was unable to follow his usual practice of removing the musket balls or shrapnel from gunshot wounds. Four Frenchmen hid for 4 days after being injured and one British soldier was captured and imprisoned for a fortnight; with only light bandages, all wounds healed promptly. As with Paré, Hunter recognized the value of this unintended experiment and he no longer operated routinely to remove all fragments. He learned that

> balls when obliged to be left, seldom or ever did any harm when at rest, and when not in a vital part; for balls have been known to lie in the body for years, and are often never found at all, and yet the person has found no inconvenience. [Hunter, 1794]

Tradition Clouded Reasoning

Many therapies were never tested but were trustfully accepted; consequently, treatments such as bleeding and blistering persisted for centuries. A simple trial would have readily exposed their ineffectiveness and harmfulness to patients. Unfortunately, as late as the 19th century, basic therapy still consisted of bleeding, purging, blistering, and administering salts of heavy metals (May, 1977).

James Lind (1716–1794)

One of the earliest documentations of a prospective, planned experiment was that by James Lind. During his lifetime, scurvy ravaged the crews of most sailing vessels on prolonged voyages, sometimes causing the deaths of three-quarters of the men. Lind reported the following:

> On the 20th of May 1747, I took 12 patients in the scurvy, on board the Salisbury at sea. Their cases were as similar as I could have them. . . . They lay together in one place . . . [and] had one diet common to all. . . . Two of these were ordered a quart of cyder a-day. Two others took twenty-five gutts [drops] of Elixir vitriol [aromatic sulfuric acid] three times a-day. . . . Two others took two spoonfuls of vinegar three times a-day. Two of the worst patients . . . were put under a course of sea water. Two others had each two oranges and one lemon given them every day. . . . The two remaining patients took the bigness of a nutmeg three times a-day an electuary recommended by a hospital-surgeon.
>
> The consequence was, that the most sudden and visible good effects were perceived from the use of the oranges and lemons; one of those who had taken them, being at the end of six days fit for duty. . . . The other . . . being now deemed pretty well, was appointed nurse to the rest of the sick. [Lind, 1753]

The two men assigned to drink cider seemed slightly improved, but the illness progressed in all of the other participants. Lind's trial provided a definitive cure as well as a prophylactic against scurvy. Long-established custom, however, clouded his reasoning, and he continued to recommend "change of air" as the primary therapeutic measure. Nevertheless, his narrative leaves no doubt that he recognized the necessity of uniformity regarding the characteristics of trial subjects. He tried to limit the variables to one—the treatment accorded each pair of sailors.

Because citrus fruit is subject to spoilage, Lind advised putting fresh juice in an earthen vessel and placing the vessel in a pan of water. The water was to be heated "almost to a boil" for several hours until the

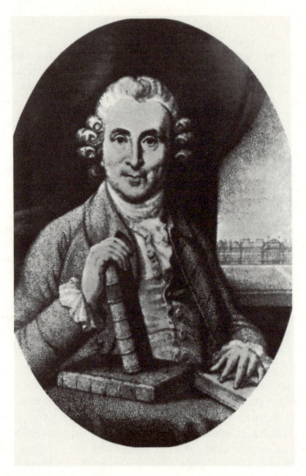

James Lind. (From Lind, J., *Treatise on Scurvy*, frontispiece, reprinted 1953. Courtesy of Edinburgh University.)

juice was the consistency of an oil or syrup. It was then to be corked and could thus be preserved and stored on ships for several years. We have since learned that vitamin C is destroyed by heat. His recipe, used as a dietary supplement, would not have cured any cases of scurvy, but we do not know whether it was ever put to the test.

The British navy did not stock lemons on its ships at sea until 1795 (Drummond and Wilbraham, 1940; Meinert, 1986).

Unbiased Recording of Data

John Haygarth (1740–1827)

John Haygarth could have fulfilled any statistician's requirements for participation in a modern clinical trial. He wrote:

> Since the year 1767, I have constantly recorded, in the patient's chamber, a full and accurate account of every important symptom, the remedies which were employed, and, when an opportunity offered, the effects which they produced. [Haygarth, 1805]

He included tables summarizing his 35-year experience with 170 patients having acute rheumatism. For each patient, the charts listed sex, age, date of first visit, date disease began, cause, latent period, prior diseases, present symptoms, joints and muscles involved, pain or swelling, chills or sweats, urinalysis, blood examination, prior remedies tried, each treatment used and effect produced, and whether the patient recovered, continued to suffer, or died. He included, in addition, a compendium in which he classified patients by age, month during which rheumatism began, month of first visit, latent period (time between exposure to cold and onset of fever), diseases that preceded or accompanied rheumatism, pulse, and groups of joints and muscles inflamed.

His evidence showed clearly that use of cinchona (Peruvian bark, Jesuits' bark) gave the best results, and he systematically worked out the optimal dosage. His detailed, concise recording would be a credit to any of our present-day studies.

Haygarth also described a small clinical trial, the results of which dealt a fatal blow to the popular use of Perkin's tractors. These metal rods were promoted for the cure of diverse diseases supposedly by some conjectured electrical influence. They were prescribed by prominent physicians, including Nathan Smith, the founder of Yale Medical

School. After Haygarth used imitation tractors on five patients, four had relief of their symptoms. The following day, he repeated the procedure on the same patients with genuine tractors and achieved identical results (Haygarth, 1801; Bull, 1959). His experiment was a good example of the placebo effect, as well as of the technique of using a patient as his own control.

William Withering (1741–1799)

Another illustration of the latter technique was provided in William Withering's *An Account of the Foxglove* (1785). He studied various preparations of digitalis in 163 patients over 10 years, and his account of the methods used to establish the best dosage constitutes a medical classic. He compared the outcome of each patient with the person's previous condition and physical status after digitalis was discontinued. Withering's unbiased inclusion of all patients receiving the drug was far ahead of most studies of his day. He believed:

> It would have been an easy task to have given select cases, whose successful treatment would have spoken strongly in favor of the medicine, and perhaps been flattering to my own reputation. But Truth and Science would condemn the procedure. I have therefore mentioned every case in which I have prescribed the Foxglove, proper or improper, successful or otherwise. Such a conduct will lay me open to the censure of those who are disposed to censure, but it will meet the approbation of others, who are the best qualified to be judges. [Withering, 1785]

Statistics Introduced into Medicine

Smallpox

Smallpox had challenged physicians since ancient times and offered one of the first opportunities for those in medicine to create a vaccine and to catalog their findings.

> Long before the eighteenth century, the Chinese had discovered a means of protecting themselves against smallpox: they blew the powdered scabs that had fallen from the skin of an infected person into the nostrils of a healthy one. In Turkey and Greece it was common practice to prick the skin in three different places with a

needle that had previously been pushed into a fresh smallpox pustule. [Taton, 1963]

This latter procedure was called "variolation" and was introduced in Britain around 1718, arousing interest in comparing the relative risk in natural cases with that in the new procedure. During the Boston epidemic of 1721, the American clergyman Cotton Mather (1663–1728) reported before the Royal Society that more than 1 in 6 of all who acquired the disease in the natural fashion died but that of 300 inoculated, only about 1 in 60 died. During that period in London, 1 of 6 natural cases, but only 1 of 91 inoculated cases, proved fatal (Shryock, 1979). These determinations required only simple calculations, but "for the first time, a mathematical procedure involving something more than ordinary measurement was employed in the service of medicine" (Shryock, 1979). As techniques improved, such analyses developed greater significance.

Daniel Bernoulli, an eminent member of the distinguished Bernoulli family, published an essay (Bernoulli, 1766) in which he described an expanded analysis of smallpox mortality. He calculated the risk of death and the life expectancy at different ages in both the natural and induced disease (Shryock, 1979).

In 1798, Edward Jenner's treatise on cowpox vaccination was published. This would have offered an ideal opportunity for a planned trial because many persons who had had cowpox were available, there were cases of active smallpox, and there was no shortage of volunteers desiring vaccinations. The early studies, however, created confusion and distrust of the vaccine.

Jenner (1749–1823) initially described 14 people who had had cowpox in the past, sometimes many decades earlier; none got smallpox from subsequent inoculation with matter from an active smallpox lesion. Ten different persons were intentionally infected with cowpox virus and four of these were later challenged with inoculation of the contents of a pustule from a patient with active smallpox. None contracted smallpox (Jenner, 1798). This appeared to be an explicit positive result for vaccination, but it did not prove to be so definitive (Bull, 1959). Jenner's evidence was sparse, his vaccine strains were not available for wide use, and it was feared that the artificial protection would not be effective against the naturally occurring smallpox.

The first large trial was inaugurated in London the year following Jenner's publication. The study was carried out in the Smallpox and

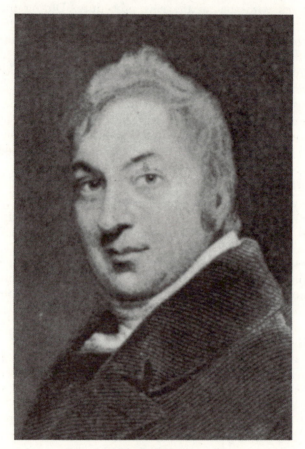

Edward Jenner.

Inoculation Hospital and was started with matter taken from an infected cow. Two-thirds of the participants, however, developed small-pox about the time they were vaccinated. This vaccine was distributed widely in Britain and abroad. There were many arguments about true and spurious cowpox vaccines, about the accurate identity of the viruses in the original vaccines, about the possibility of transmitting syphilis by vaccination, and, especially, about who should get the credit for developing a successful vaccine (Baxby, 1981).

These trials never fulfilled their promise, probably because investigators of that era had no knowledge about viruses, observations and techniques were variable, and the true diagnosis of the patient from whom Jenner's vaccine originated was in doubt (Baxby, 1981, pp. 105–17). The process of vaccination, however, was a success, and in 1958 Ingraham wrote, "In the course of the 161 years since Jenner's discovery, it has probably saved as many lives throughout the world as all the rest of preventive and curative medicine."

The world had to wait almost 100 years for a well-planned prospective vaccine trial, which was conducted by Pasteur in his quest for an anthrax prophylaxis (see Chapter 2). In contrast to Jenner, Pasteur had a background of sound scientific knowledge, the trial was well conducted, and a stunningly conclusive result was achieved.

The smallpox epidemics, however, did stimulate the registration of vital statistics. Officials in many European towns had started preserving vital records during the 16th century. Lists of deaths were sometimes published weekly and, particularly during an outbreak of small-pox, residents who had the means left town when the number of deaths began to rise (Shryock, 1979).

Demographic Statistics

Counting Heads

Statistical data were recorded in very early times. Before undertaking the construction of the pyramids, about 3050 B.C., the Egyptians compiled information concerning population and wealth, and there are accounts of statistical works in China that date to as early as 2300 B.C. Two enumerations of the Israelites are mentioned in the book of Numbers, and a census was taken in Greece for the purpose of levying taxes in 594 B.C. The Romans not only counted their people but also prepared surveys of the entire country and recorded births and deaths; they required registration of all citizens and inventories of their possessions as a basis for taxation.

After the fall of the Roman Empire, however, many centuries passed before other governments established systems for collecting official facts and figures; very few statistical records of value were made during the Middle Ages (Pollock, 1953).

Sir William Petty (1623–1687)

Sir William Petty and John Graunt were friends and colleagues during the mid-1600s, and both were pioneers in the field of vital and medical statistics. Petty abandoned a naval career to study medicine at the universities of Leiden, Paris, and Oxford. He was, in turn, a physician, professor of anatomy at Oxford, a musician, inventor, surveyor and landowner in Ireland, and a member of Parliament, but "whether he could fairly be called a mathematician is doubtful" (Greenwood, 1941).

> From 1655 to 1656, Petty undertook a survey of Ireland as a basis for the distribution of forfeited lands to army officers and soldiers, and he also became a member of the commission that distributed the lands. Petty himself took over a great deal of land and was later charged with dishonesty, which led to many lawsuits. By the end of his appointment in 1659, the initially poor university professor had become a great landowner and a wealthy man. [Hald, 1990]

He was one of the founders of the Royal Society of London for the Improvement of Natural Knowledge (1660) and an initiator of political arithmetic, which he defined as the art of reasoning by figures upon things relating to government. His most significant work was his *Treatise on Taxes and Contributions*.

Petty proposed the organization of a central statistical office that would accumulate an extraordinary abundance of information. The census would include births, marriages, deaths, occupations, the number of houses and housekeepers, the number of hearths, the number of statute acres, the number of people by sex and age group (those under 10 years, between 10 and 70, and over 70; males aged 16 to 60; and females between 16 and 48 and how many of these women were married), how many persons were incurable impotents, and how many lived on alms.

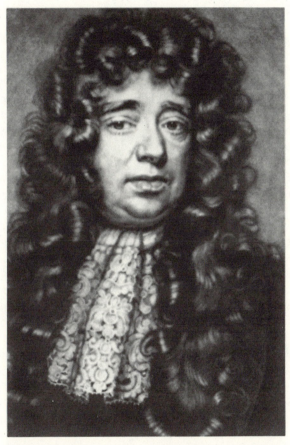

Sir William Petty. (From Keynes, G., 1971, *A Bibliography of Sir William Petty FRS and of Observations on the Bills of Mortality by John Graunt FRS*, frontispiece. Copyright © 1971, Oxford University Press, Courtesy of Oxford University Press.)

Petty offered many suggestions about how to use the data file. For example, he states:

> The numbers of people that are of every yeare old from one to 100, and the number of them that dye at every such yeare's age, do shew to how many yeare's value the life of any person of any age is equivalent and consequently makes a Par between the value of the Estates [state or condition] for life and for yeares. [Greenwood, 1941]

In Greenwood's opinion, this is the most remarkable sentence that Petty wrote, for it "suggests that he had grasped the principle of an accurate life table, viz., a survivorship table based upon a knowledge of rates of mortality in age groups" (Greenwood, 1941). No such table was constructed from population data until the end of the 18th century because data of the age distribution of the living population were not obtained until then.

After extensive study of Petty's life and writings, Greenwood (1941) concluded that Petty had a somewhat careless, happy-go-lucky attitude and that his psychological makeup would predict him to be an innovator, "directing attention to a number of problems that deserved study, but not leading to the production of any solid contribution to knowledge."

Statisticians, however, should commend him for his plan for a central statistical office. Petty recorded his definite, detailed scheme with schedules for each parish 150 years before the General Register Office came into being (Greenwood, 1941).

"When one passes, [however], from what Petty suggested to what he actually did himself, our praise must be qualified" (Greenwood, 1941).

Apparently, Petty understood the components that need to be included in a life table, but it is questionable whether he comprehended the necessary calculations. "Whether Petty also realized that under certain conditions a life table could be constructed without knowledge of the ages of the living population is a controversial matter" (Greenwood, 1941).

Petty used some of Graunt's methods and results, but Petty's *Papers* (1755) did not equal the quality of Graunt's statistical book. In fact, some of Petty's statements are quite erroneous, as in "Tis four times more likely that one of 16 yeares old should live to be 70, than a new born Babe." Although there is no life table for England in 1674, if the

Liverpool table by Farr (1871) is applied, the chance would be double the infant's chance, not four times as large (Greenwood, 1941).

Armitage, however, wrote that Petty had no doubt about the power of statistics:

> God send me the use of things, and notions, whose foundations are secure and the superstructures mathematical reasoning; for want of which props so many Governments doe reel and stagger. [Petty, year unknown; Armitage, 1984]

John Graunt (1620–1674)

A man of one book, John Graunt described his statistical research in *Natural and Political Observations Made Upon the London Bills of Mortality* (1662) and taught us that "very imperfect data, if patiently considered, will tell us something it is good for us to know" (Greenwood, 1942). While active as a young merchant, he began to study the death records that had been kept by London parishes since 1532. Graunt was the first person to recognize that numerical data on human populations warranted more than a passing glance (Sutherland, 1963).

> Data for the Bills were gathered by searchers, who were generally elderly women, usually susceptible to bribes, ignorant of medicine, and often a bit intoxicated. Their assignment was to investigate and report the deaths and quarantine the diseased. The searchers reported their findings to Parish Clerks on Tuesdays, and by 10:00 A.M. Thursdays copies were issued for public sale. [Kargon, 1963]

Graunt explained his interest:

> Having been born and bred in the city of London, and having always observed, that most of them who constantly took in the weekly Bills of Mortality, made little other use of them, than to look at the foot, how the Burials increased and decreased; and among the Casualties, what had happened rare and extraordinary in the week current: so as they might take the same as a Text to talk upon in the next Company; and withall in the Plague-time how the sickness increased or decreased, that so the Rich might judge of the necessity of their removall, and Tradesmen might conjecture what doings they were like to have in their respective dealings.
>
> Now I thought that the Wisdome of our City had certainly designed the laudable practice of takeing and distributing these Accompts, for other and greater uses than those above mentioned,

or at least some other uses might be made of them. [Graunt, 1662, p. 17; Kargon, 1963]

For data covering more than 60 years, the only figures Graunt had available to him were the numbers of males and females christened and buried and the causes of death. For the latter, data were listed under 60 headings. He classified death rates according to the causes of death, among which he included overpopulation, and noted that the metropolitan death rate exceeded that in the farming communities. Although the male birth rate was higher than the female, it was balanced by a greater mortality rate for males, so that the population was divided almost evenly. For variation, he collected data from outlying areas as well as from London proper.

He continually assessed the trustworthiness of his information, judged his sources, and accepted no statement that he had a means of testing. He questioned why a particular diagnosis was being reported more frequently as a cause of death (syphilis, rickets) and tried, as far as possible, to verify these reports. After extensive work in London hospitals, he learned to group together multiple diagnoses that likely represented one disease (livergrown, spleen, and rickets in children).

Graunt did not know the ages of the dead. To estimate the percentage of children dying before the age of 6 years, he selected from the list of causes of death those illnesses that he thought struck only children not more than 4 or 5 years old. He chose thrush, convulsions, rickets, teeth and worms, abortives, chrysomes, infants, livergrown, and overlaid. These gave him some 70,000 child deaths out of about 229,000 total deaths. Then he assigned one-half of the deaths from smallpox, swinepox, measles, and worms without convulsions also to children under 6 years and reached the final conclusion that about "36% of all quick conceptions die before six years old" (Greenwood, 1942).

Was this a reasonable determination? More than 200 years later, William Farr published a life table for London, using knowledge of the numbers and ages of the living population. Interpolating in that, Greenwood found that about 32% of quick conceptions died before 6 years old.

Perhaps Graunt's most important innovation was the life table based on survival, although it appeared as a minor insertion in his book. Using two rates of survivorship (to ages 6 and 76) derived from actual observations, he predicted the percentage of persons who would live to each successive age and their life expectancy year by year. After detailed analysis, Greenwood (1942) concluded that "it is evident that Graunt was not at all clear in his mind as to how to use a life-table." The table, as well as some of his other calculations, contains many errors, but he and Petty were far ahead of their contemporaries in demographic statistics.

Graunt was awarded recognition during his lifetime. Within 2 weeks of the publication of his book, he was nominated for fellowship in the Royal Society, allegedly on the special recommendation of King Charles II (Sprat, 1722; Kargon, 1963). In a tercentenary tribute to Graunt, Sutherland (1963) wrote:

> I believe it is fair to claim that few of the developments in statistics since his time would really have surprised Graunt. Certainly in the descriptive field we can claim little more than numerical refinement; more accurate nomenclature and enumeration, population censuses, standard deviations and correlation coefficients have merely given numerical form to concepts he grasped without their assistance. Even the most important single step in the advance of statistics, the marriage of descriptive analysis to the theory of probability, would not, I believe, have disconcerted Graunt. He was, I have suggested, aware of the existence of chance variation, and understood probability levels; he would surely have welcomed this additional weapon for discriminating between reasonable and unreasonable inferences from his data. . . .
>
> The other major development in statistics, that of experimental design, would not strike Graunt as wholly strange either, in view of his attempt to obtain a geographically scattered sample of parish records for study.

Edmund Halley (1656–1742)

Using the death records of Breslau for the period 1687 to 1691, Edmund Halley created the first mortality tables of great importance. He presented his paper, *An Estimate of the Degrees of Mortality of Mankind, drawn from curious Tables of the Births and Funerals at the City of Breslaw; with an Attempt to ascertain the Price of Annuities on Lives*, in 1693 (Hald, 1990). While Petty and Graunt did not know the ages of the deceased, the bills of mortality at Breslau supplied the ages and sex of all who died during each month as well as the number of births. The population size was still missing (Hald, 1990).

Halley attempted to relate mortality and age to a population and

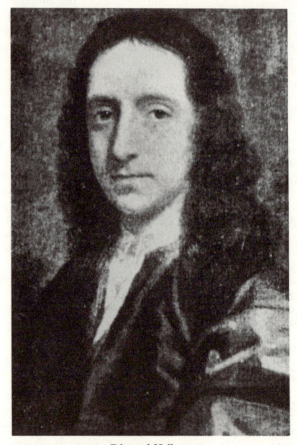

Edmund Halley.

thereby influenced the future development of actuarial tables in life insurance. He wrote that

> the Purchaser ought to pay for only such a part of the value of the Annuity, that he has Chances that he is living; and this ought to be computed yearly, and the Sum of all those yearly values being added together, will amount to the value of the Annuity for the Life of the Person proposed. [Halley, 1693; Hald, 1990, p. 139]

Halley's scientific reputation stems primarily from his work in astronomy. As a young man, he left Oxford without taking his degree and went to the island of St. Helena to observe the stars that were too near the south pole to be visible in Europe. He was elected a fellow of the Royal Society at the age of 22 on the basis of his catalog of the positions of 341 southern stars (Hald, 1990, p. 132). Applying Newton's theory, he figured out the orbits of 24 comets.

> Noting that the orbits of the comets of 1531, 1607, and 1682 were similar, he conjectured that these comets were one and the same object moving periodically in an elliptical orbit, and he predicted the next appearance of this comet, today known as Halley's comet. [Hald, 1990, p. 132]

We can all take comfort from knowing that Sir Isaac Newton once told Halley that lunar theory "made his head ache and kept him awake so often that he would think of it no more" (Berry, 1898; Stigler, 1986).

Halley never again addressed the problems of life tables, annuities, or demographic statistics, and Hald (1990) stated that "it is a singular proof of his versatility that he produced this seminal paper in a field rather far from his main interests."

Creating the Life Table

Petty, Graunt, Halley, and many other mathematicians and statisticians contributed to the development of the life table. Petty was primarily interested in economics, and many of his *Papers* (1755) presented a more focused concern with political issues rather than statistics. Clearly, however, both Petty and Graunt understood that their studies and publications had a direct connection or relationship to public health and to medicine in general.

Greenwood (1942) believed that Halley certainly perceived the flaws in Graunt's life table and also quickly grasped the commercial importance of the life table for the insurance business. For 150 years after Graunt's death, very little was done to improve the life table and medical statistics.

> Down to 1801 the population as a whole had not been counted, forty years more passed before a reasonable age distribution was secured, and it was thirty-eight years after the first denominator (populations) that the first numerator (deaths) of the fundamental fraction was obtained. [Greenwood, 1942]

Accumulating Knowledge of Probability

The study of probability was an outgrowth of gambling. We do not know when men first started to play games of chance, but by 1400 B.C. dice existed in Egypt. Shortly thereafter, the dots came to be arranged in the patterns that we still use today (David, 1955). We know this because it is quite usual to find several sets of dice, ". . . some untampered and others obviously loaded" in the burial chambers of Egyptian kings (Neyman, 1976).

The earliest documentation of counting the number of ways three dice can fall appears to have occurred in a Latin poem presumably written between A.D. 1220 and 1250 (Kendall, 1956). Dice led to other games for the people of the 17th century, who seemed to enjoy creating or solving problems based on dice, cards, roulette wheels, or the toss of coins. A typical problem of this period was Gambler's Ruin. Two players, Peter and Paul, toss a coin. For each head, Paul pays Peter $1; for each tail, Peter pays Paul $1. If Peter initially has "a" dollars and Paul has "b" dollars, what is the probability that Peter will be ruined? The probability is equal to $b/(a + b)$, the proportion of the total capital initially in Paul's possession (*Encyclopaedia Britannica Micropaedia*, 15th ed., 9:714, 1985).

In 1657, Christiaan Huygens (1629–1695), a Dutch physicist better known for his work on lenses, visited France and found that the French mathematicians were very interested in the principles of chances. Huygens worked out a theory of chances, and the Latin translation of his efforts (1657) was probably the first book published on the calculus of probabilities (Kendall, 1956). By the mid-1700s, the calculus of probabilities had been formalized and was a topic of common discourse among mathematicians, who for the most part were no longer amateurs like their 17th century counterparts, but who were almost exclusively professionals—university professors and members of scientific academies (Taton, 1963, pp. 397–424). These 18th century mathematicians naturally applied their wisdom to the new subject, and some in particular deserve a place in history for their original thinking.

Thomas Bayes (1702–1761)

During his lifetime, the Rev. Thomas Bayes wrote *Divine Benevolence, or an Attempt to Prove That the Principal End of the Divine Providence and Government is the Happiness of His Creatures* (1731) and *An Introduction to the Doctrine of Fluxions, and a Defence of the Mathematicians Against the Objections of the Author of The Analyst* (1736), which opposed attacks on the mathematical logic of Newton's calculus. But it is for "An Essay towards Solving a Problem in the Doctrine of Chances," found after his death and mailed by his friend Richard Price (1723–1791) to the Royal Society, that Bayes has a permanent niche in the scientific hall of fame. In this essay, Bayes presented a theorem that provided a way to predict a possible future outcome with knowledge of past experience—to ascertain the probability of an event from earlier observations. Briefly, he theorized that "*Given* the number of times in which an unknown event has happened and failed: *Required* the chance that the probability of its happening in a single trial lies somewhere between any two degrees of probability that can be named" (Bayes, 1763). He then presented ten propositions of probability or chance and their mathematical explanations.

Before the publication of Bayes's dissertation, mathematicians determined probabilities only when they knew the prior state of things. Bayes's postulate supplied a mathematical means by which a statistician could allocate various values to the unknowns in a problem in light of previous works or established beliefs, enabling the statistician to make educated estimates. Further, as statisticians accumulate data to answer questions or hypotheses, they can alter their estimates to reflect the actual data (Reid, 1982). This method is called *inverse probability*—a term first used by Laplace (Peters, 1987).

Pierre-Simon de Laplace (1749–1827)

Bayes's *Essay* (1763) did not receive wide attention, and many mathematicians of that period were probably unaware of the man and his ideas until around 1780 (Stigler, 1986, p. 103). The principle that is known today as the Bayes theorem was formulated by Laplace in 1774;

thus, we must ask "Where did Laplace get his principle? The statement and approach were so different from those of Bayes that we can discount the possibility that Laplace had seen Bayes's essay" (Stigler, 1986, p. 103). And yet, using the same premise as Bayes, Laplace suggested ways in which the theorem could be applied to demographic studies and to a large number of scientific questions. With his work, probability theory may be said to have become an independent branch of mathematics (Taton, 1963, pp. 397–424). When Laplace published his classic study *Théorie Analytique des Probabilités* in 1812, he mentioned the potential for using some of these statistical techniques in medical research. Usually, it is supposed that Laplace first applied the theorem to determine the probability that the sun will rise tomorrow, but that is one of the illustrations given in the first issue of Bayes's monograph in 1763 (K. Pearson, 1978).

Although the explanation and delineation of the theorem may have been explicitly clear to Laplace, it has been subjected to many interpretations and connotations by mathematicians and other scientists whose viewpoints of the Bayesian method differ. Laplace described probability as follows.

> The probability of an event is equal to the sum of each favorable case multiplied by its probability, divided by the sum of the products of each possible case multiplied by its probability, and if each case is equally probable, the probability of the event is equal to the number of favorable cases divided by the number of all possible cases. [Grattan-Guinness, 1978]

Thus, the Bayesian approach allows one to predict the probability of any occurrence, even if it is a single event, such as the probability of a declaration of war. On the other hand, the "frequentist" reasoning allows for the designation of probabilities and confidence intervals for situations or events in experiments that hypothetically have the possibility of many repetitions (Reid, 1982, p. 24).

In recent years, Bayes's theorem has been used in setting up computer software programs to help with medical diagnosis and with the design and analysis of clinical trials.

> Knowledge of the frequency of a particular symptom constellation in each of k possible diseases, coupled with knowledge of the relative frequency of each of the k diagnoses in the population at hand, permits one to determine, with the use of Bayes' theorem, the likelihood of a diagnosis if a patient presents with the symptom

complex. In this way, given the symptoms, the most probable diagnosis . . . can be determined. [Colton, 1974]

Daniel Bernoulli (1700–1782)

Daniel Bernoulli was a Swiss physicist and mathematician who not only published the early skilled analysis of smallpox mortality already mentioned but also wrote eight memoirs that contained major contributions to probability theory. He used differential equations systematically to derive a number of formulas, raised the problem of testing statistical assumptions, and studied random processes (Sheynin, 1977). His memoir on maximum likelihood or the most probable choice between several discrepant observations (Bernoulli, 1777) was considered by Kendall (1961) to be remarkably in advance of its time.

The Bernoulli family produced nine distinguished scholars, remembered primarily for their contributions to mathematics, although they excelled in many other areas of science. Daniel was a doctor of medicine as well as a professor of anatomy, botany, and philosophy. During his lifetime, he received more than ten awards from the Academy of Paris, and he and his father shared a prize as coauthors of an essay on the reasons for the various inclinations in the orbits of planets. Daniel created a statistical test of randomness of these orbits.

The Bernoulli family tree has been recorded, but only the males are listed—not a word about mothers, wives, or sisters. "This makes it impossible to understand how this remarkable strain petered out" (K. Pearson, 1978, pp. 221–22).

The doctrine of *moral fortune* (*Encyclopaedia Britannica*, 11th ed. 22:386, 1911) was first expressed by Daniel with reference to the famous Petersburg Paradox, so called because it first appeared in the commentaries of the Petersburg Academy (Bernoulli, 1738a; Westergaard, 1968). In the Petersburg Paradox, player A receives a fee from anyone who desires to play the game. Player B pays and then tosses a coin in the air. If head appears at the first throw, the tosser receives a shilling from A. If tail appears, the tosser throws the coin again and gets two shillings if head appears on the second throw. If the tosser loses the second time, he plays again and is entitled to four shillings if head appears on the third throw, etc. Whenever tail appears, the payment to player B is doubled. Thus, the question is: what is a fair charge for player B to enter the game? Calculation of the fee should be based on the expected amount that player A would pay if the coin were fair.

One aspect of the Petersburg Paradox is the calculation of the chance of a win at each throw, which is obviously one-half to throw a head for each toss of a fair coin. Another aspect concerns the expected amount of the payout for player A. Because there is a finite chance of an infinitely long series of tails followed by a head (even with a fair coin), A's expectation is to pay out an infinite amount of money. Consequently, the only fair fee for player B is an infinite amount of money! For an apparently very simple game, there is a very high probability (more than 0.99) that player A will pay out a finite amount of money; but because there is an infinitesimal chance of an infinitely long series of consecutive tails followed by a head, then A, by the rules of calculating expectations, should expect to pay out an infinite amount of money!

George-Louis Leclerc de Buffon (1777) stated that there would not be time during a whole life for playing more than a certain number of games (Westergaard, 1968). In 1761, Jean Le Rond d'Alembert "maintained that if tail arrives three times in succession it is more likely that head will be shown next time than tail, and the oftener the tail arrives successively the greater will be the chance of head at the next throw. In this way he can easily find a solution which gives the player a finite expectation" (Westergaard, 1968). The statement by d'Alembert is incorrect for fair coins; if tail appears many more times than head, one suspects either a "loaded" coin or that the coin is being tossed so that it spins in a repeating pattern each time.

Some mathematicians and philosophers dwelled on the moral implications of the problem and discussed how soon one of the players would be ruined (*Encyclopaedia Britannica*, 11th ed. **22**:386, 1911).

The Petersburg Paradox is a precursor of the doubling-down system used by gamblers today: if a bet is made with approximately a 50% chance of a win on the turn of a roulette wheel (e.g., a bet for red), the gambler doubles his stake with each subsequent turn of the wheel if he loses, so that he ultimately realizes a profit if he wins on some turn. This doubling-down strategy has a high probability of a win in the short run; ultimately, however, it will be a losing tactic. Unfortunately, there is a finite chance of a long series of losses (e.g., a long run of black on the roulette wheel), so that the amount to be wagered on the following turn exceeds either the bet limit of the gambling house or the stake of the gambler.

Astronomy, statistics, and gambling are not the only fields to which Daniel Bernoulli made contributions; he was a physicist and *Hydrodynamica* (1738b), his paramount publication, includes descriptions of certain hydraulic principles that later came to be known as Bernoulli's Law. This Law explains many of our familiar phenomena. A baseball thrown forward with a spin will follow a curved path, determined by Bernoulli's Law. An airplane flies because the air flowing over the wing has a higher velocity than the air flowing under the wing, and the pressure on top of the wing is thereby reduced. The Law shows that the pressure is greater where the velocity is least. This difference in pressure causes the plane to lift (Chow, 1966). Bernoulli's kinetic theory of gases was outlined in *Hydrodynamica*, and one of the principles delineated was applied to the development of the modern carburetor for the internal-combustion engine.

The 18th century could rightfully be labeled the golden age of mathematics because many creative scientists from various countries (France, Germany, Switzerland, Italy, England, and Belgium) published original contributions that served to advance the discipline by leaps and bounds. We have described briefly the works of Bayes, Laplace, and Bernoulli because of their later applications in medical trials. Other mathematicians of this period (Abraham deMoivre, Carl Friedrich Gauss, Siméon-Denis Poisson) made contributions to statistics although their predominant work was in other areas.

deMoivre was a French mathematician who moved to London after the revocation of the Edict of Nantes and became a teacher. It is judged that he was the first to become aware of "normal distribution." He wrote *The Doctrine of Chances, or a Method of Calculating the Probabilities of Events at Play* (1718). Edmond Hoyle appears to have learned probability by studying the book. In the mid-1700s, Hoyle wrote several volumes on games and lotteries, outlining accepted rules, strategies for play, and probability calculations for various situations (Bellhouse, 1993). Even today, we play many of our card games and use gambling tactics "according to Hoyle." Bellhouse's research showed that from the early 16th to the mid-18th centuries, most of the English literature on gambling centered around cheating. False dice, sleight of hand, and methods of shuffling were the focus of many books. Contrary to a sustained belief, gambling may not have actuated probability theories; in fact, the development of probability calculus seemed to give impetus to the creation of plans or methods of play for card games, games of chance, and for betting or wagering.

Poisson, also French, is famous for his applications of mathematics to electricity, magnetism, and mechanics. He was one of the founders of the theory of elasticity, studying stresses and strains and the mathematics of small displacements within a medium in a state of stress (Deimel, 1953). In statistics, his name is attached to the Poisson distribution, an important work on probability. If the probability (*p*) of an event at each trial is very small, but the number (*n*) of trials is large enough that *np* approaches a constant value of small to moderate size, then the number of events observed follows a Poisson distribution.

Gauss was a German mathematician who worked primarily in astronomy and surveying. In statistics, he is known for his ideas on errors of observation and for Gaussian distribution, the graph of which is the typical bell-shaped normal curve.

Statistics Comes of Age

Since Graunt's innovative work on the analysis of vital statistics, many researchers have investigated such data. It was not until around 1800, however, that this sphere of work began to be called *statistics* (Hald, 1990, p. 82). The first to use the word *statistik* was Gottfried Achenwall (1719–1772), a professor of philosophy at the University of Göttingen (Pollock, 1953). The word comes from the Italian *statista* (statesman) or *stato* (state) and was used in Italy in the 16th century to describe facts of interest to a statesman; that meaning for the word gradually disappeared around the beginning of the 19th century (Hald, 1990, pp. 81–82).

Lambert Adolphe Jacques Quetelet (1796–1874)

A primary advance of the scientific method in statistical study resulted because astronomers required some way of making correct determinations from their voluminous array of observational data.

> It was found that errors of observation were symmetrically grouped about their arithmetic mean, where they were clustered most closely, and decreasing continuously and equally in number in accordance with a certain law, called the normal law of errors, as the observation receded in either direction from the mean. This law, also known as the Law of Probability or the Law of Chance, was found by the great Belgian astronomer and mathematician, Jacques Quetelet, to govern not merely the distribution of errors of measurement of inanimate things, or direct the action of "blind chance,"

such as the manner in which coins, when tossed, turn up "heads" or "tails," but also the chance distributions in the animate world. [Engberg, 1953]

Early in the 19th century, Quetelet devoted the major part of his career to the study of statistics. When Belgium took its first census in 1829, Quetelet analyzed the data and made noteworthy observations on the influence of age, sex, occupation, and economic condition (Pollock, 1953). In a distinguished treatise, he applied methods of averages and probabilities to man and focused on "the average man":

> The greater the number of individuals observed, the more do individual peculiarities, whether physical or moral, become effaced, and allow the general facts to predominate, by which society exists and is preserved. [Quetelet, 1835, with translation in 1842; Stigler, 1986, p. 172]

Quetelet was involved in the formation of the Statistical Society of London, which later became the Royal Statistical Society. He had traveled to London in 1833 as the delegate from Belgium to a meeting of the British Association for the Advancement of Science. He brought with him a collection of data on crime that he intended to present. He found, however, that there was no suitable section of the association before whom he could appear.

Several interested men met with Quetelet in a private room to hear his statistics, and, although chastised by the association for irregularity, they were allowed to petition for the creation of a new section. Cochran (1982) wrote that one of the considerations was to decide whether statistics was a branch of science. The members decided that as long as statisticians limited their sphere to the acquisition, cataloging, and presentation of data, that was science. If statisticians began interpreting findings, that would be "argumentation, with passions and politics entering, and that was not science."

Florence David (1984) explained why the statisticians readily accepted this limitation:

> The idea that the new society should confine itself to "numerical facts, systematically collected" may seem strange to us but it was very much in keeping with the climate of the time. For instance, in 1835 a committee of the French Academy of Sciences reported against any numerical method in medicine, "for each patient has his own individuality, problems in medicine are always individual, the facts presenting themselves for solution one by one, the treatment

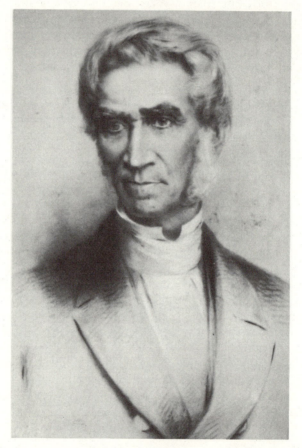

Lambert Adolphe Jacques Quetelet. (From Rosenbaum, S., 1984, The growth of the Royal Statistical Society. *J R Stat Soc A* **147**:377. Courtesy of the Royal Statistical Society.)

in each case depending on a happy instinct supported by numerous comparisons and guided by experience."

A section dealing with statistics was duly established, but the following year the members of this enterprising group voted to create a separate Statistical Society (I. D. Hill, 1984).

It is of interest to note that Quetelet was also a tutor of Queen Victoria's husband, Prince Albert. The Prince must have learned his lessons in statistics well because, in 1861, he presided over the founding of the International Statistical Institute (Kendall, 1972).

The Early Use of Statistics to Evaluate Therapy

Vaccination against smallpox became an established and widely practiced procedure after the early 1800s, and the statistical studies of inoculation ceased. Interest in statistics, however, had been aroused, and even before the turn of the century it occurred to people that statistical techniques could be used to measure the value of a treatment.

Rush versus Cobbett

In 1793, Philadelphia was experiencing a severe outbreak of yellow fever, and Dr. Benjamin Rush (1745–1813) had announced his sure cure—bleeding and purging. William Cobbett (1763–1835), an English politician, requested the patients' records and proof that the treatment was effective. Since Rush had not kept complete figures, Cobbett examined the city's death notices (Shryock, 1979). Rush had begun to prescribe his cure on September 12, and on that date there were 23 deaths from yellow fever. The doctor and his team of nonmedical helpers tried to apply his "cure" to all victims of yellow fever and treated a high percentage of those afflicted. Mortality increased daily, however, rising to 56, then to 96, and, finally, to 119 on October 11. Cobbett observed that the famous cure was "one of those great discoveries which have contributed to the depopulation of the earth" (Cobbett, 1800; Shryock, 1979).

The mortality figures seemed to show a positive correlation between the increase in bleeding and purging and the increase in deaths. No mention was made, however, about investigating other variables such as the lack of treatment in some cases, alternate therapy by other physicians, or the normal curve of the epidemic (Shryock, 1979). King

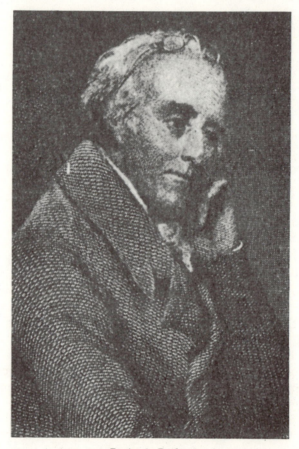

Benjamin Rush.

wrote that the amount of blood removed by Rush staggers our belief. Often within a period of 5 days, he removed more than 100 ounces, or more than 3 quarts from a patient (King, 1964).

Pierre Charles Alexandre Louis (1787–1872)

Around 1820, the physician Pierre Louis fled from Russia, unhappy and disillusioned by an epidemic of diphtheria, which, as Sir William Osler said, "struck the terror of helplessness and hopelessness into his heart" (Steiner, 1940). Louis returned to his native France, removed himself from practice, and for the next 6 years did nothing but study ward cases and autopsies in three Paris hospitals. The very number of cases at Louis's disposal may have suggested to him the method he soon adopted for analyzing his accumulated data—to list the cases in numerical form and to check the outcomes of one group receiving a certain treatment against those of another group denied it (Shryock, 1979). Louis strongly advocated the use of such methods but may not have created them. James Jackson, an American physician, stated that a numerical scheme had been employed by George Fordyce in 1793. James Jackson, Jr., whom Louis loved as a son and to whom the American translation of one of his books was dedicated, had studied with Louis but died at the age of 24 at the "very outset of a brilliant career" (Steiner, 1940). Louis, however, is credited with expanding Hippocrates's observation on the importance of seeing, touching, and hearing the patient while conducting a physical examination to include recording the information (Steiner, 1940).

After analyzing about 2000 observations that he had gathered during his six-year hiatus, Louis published eight papers before writing his celebrated *Researches on Phthisis: Anatomical, Pathological and Therapeutical* (1825), which was translated into many languages and widely disseminated.

Charles J. B. Williams (1884), a pupil of Laennec, remembered Louis:

> In the same ward, we often saw a tall solemn man with spectacles, diligently taking notes alone, not accompanying the physician. This was M. Louis, collecting materials for his elaborate work on Phthisis, which established his reputation for statistics; these he held to be the only proper basis of medicine. In that line he became famous; but he was equally remarkable for the gloominess

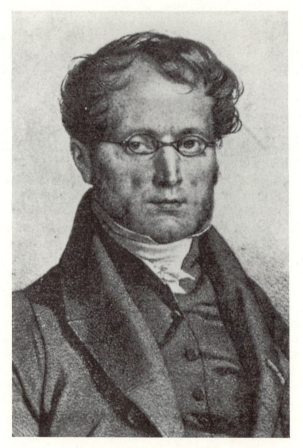

Pierre Charles Alexandre Louis.

of his predictions, and the inefficiency of his practice. [Williams, 1884; Steiner, 1940]

According to U.S. physician Elisha Bartlett (1804–1855), Louis used his numerical method (between 1821 and 1828) to study the effects of bloodletting in 50 cases of pneumonia that resolved favorably and in 28 cases that terminated in death. Of the 50 patients, 23 were bled for the first time within the first 4 days of the disease; the average duration of pain was 6 days and the average duration of the disease was 17 days. Twenty-seven of the fifty patients were bled for the first time between the fifth and ninth days of the disease; their average duration of pain was 8 days and the average duration of the disease was 20 days. Every precaution was taken to have comparable groups. Louis published the results in 1828, and, according to Bartlett, considered himself justified in concluding that "blood-letting has a favorable effect upon the march of pneumonia; that it abridges its duration; but that this effect is much less than had been generally supposed" (Bartlett, 1848).

Bartlett, however, recognized that, instead of revealing the absolute effects of bloodletting, the investigation directly showed the difference in its effects when performed early or late in the disease. He wrote that "so strong and so universal was the confidence in this remedy [bloodletting], that the feeling became very general, that it was essential to the cure of the disease; or, at least, that it could not be omitted, without the most imminent hazard to the patient" (Bartlett, 1848). Thus, Louis's incorrect conclusion about the benefits of bloodletting provides evidence that even the best of researchers can sometimes make mistakes. Bartlett excused Louis's error because of the widespread and traditional acceptance of bloodletting as a beneficial practice.

In 1834 Louis gave strict guidelines to be followed in his "numerical method" for evaluating various therapies. This appeared to be a simple process of counting the cures for each drug or method of treatment. In actual practice, however, it was neither simple nor easily managed because, as Louis wrote,

> in order that the calculations may lead to useful or true results it is not sufficient to take account of the modifying powers of the individual; it is also necessary to know with precision at what period of the disease the treatment has been commenced; and especially we ought to know the natural progress of the disease, in all its degrees, when it is abandoned to itself, and whether the subjects have or have not committed errors of regimen; with other

> particulars . . . it neither can nor ought to be applied to any other
> than exact observations, and these are not common; . . . this
> method requires much more labour and time than the most distin-
> guished members of our profession can dedicate to it. . . . The
> research of truth requires much labour, and is beset with difficulty.
> [Louis, 1834; Bull, 1959]

By 1835, when Louis published his *Researches on the Effects of
Bloodletting*, he had studied not only the 78 cases of pneumonia already
described but also

> 33 cases of erysipelas and 23 cases of inflammation of the throat. He
> concluded that there was no appreciable difference in mortality or
> in duration or type of symptoms or signs between patients bled and
> those not bled or between patients bled at different stages of the
> disease. This result, which was contrary to orthodox teaching of the
> time, caused an uproar among French physicians, but it dealt a fatal
> blow to the "depletive" treatment then in vogue. [Bull, 1959]

Louis had misgivings:

> The results of my researches on the effects of bloodletting in
> inflammation are so little in accord with the general opinion, that it
> is not without a degree of hesitation I have decided to publish them.
> After having analyzed the facts, which relate to them, for the first
> time, I thought myself deceived, and began my work anew; but
> having again from this new analysis, obtained the same results, I
> could no longer doubt their correctness. [Louis, 1836; Eisenberg,
> 1977]

He was forced to conclude:

> We infer that bloodletting has had very little influence on the
> progress of pneumonitis . . . that its influence has not been more
> evident in the cases bled copiously and repeatedly, than in those
> bled only once and to a small amount; that we do not at once arrest
> inflammations, as is too often finally imagined; that, in cases where
> it appears to be otherwise, it is undoubtedly owing, either to an
> error in diagnosis, or to the fact that the bloodletting was practiced
> at an advanced period of the disease, when it had nearly run its
> course. [Louis, 1836, p. 22; Eisenberg, 1977]

In Louis's 1836 paper he emphasized that physicians needed to
know specifically how often venesection aided and how often it im-
peded recovery. He further required that physicians' research be based
on sufficient numbers of patients and "controls" in order to eliminate

individual factors, and to establish conclusions with mathematical certainty. His was probably the first clear and emphatic realization of the value of medical statistics (Shryock, 1979).

Apparently, the main conclusion to be drawn from Louis's 1836 study is that there was essentially no difference in the mean time of the duration of symptoms or to mortality between those patients bled and those not bled. His work was certainly significant clinically, but complete data would be necessary to effect a modern statistical analysis of his numbers.

Louis, himself, later wrote:

> Medicine depends for its very existence, as a science, upon facts, and . . . truth can flow only from those that have been well and fully observed. Then and only then may a series of cases be regarded as data for the solution of a problem. . . . Accurate facts, so long as they are examined under the same points of view, must lead to identical results, no matter who be their analyser. [Louis, 1843]

Louis's recommendation is consistent with current clinical trial guidelines, one of which is "the methods of statistical analysis should be described in detail sufficient that a knowledgeable reader could reproduce the analysis if the data were available" (Simon and Wittes, 1985).

In light of his beliefs, Louis went further; in fact, he basically proposed clinical trials:

> In any epidemic, for instance, let us suppose, five hundred of the sick, *taken indiscriminately*, [are] subjected to one kind of treatment, and five hundred others, taken in the same manner, [are] treated in a different mode; if the mortality is greater among the first [five hundred] than among the second, must we not conclude that the treatment was less appropriate, or less efficacious in the first class, than in the second? . . . it is impossible to appreciate each case with mathematical exactness and it is precisely on this account that enumeration becomes necessary; by doing so, the errors (which are inevitable) being the same in both groups of patients subjected to different treatments, mutually compensate each other and they may be disregarded without sensibly affecting the exactness of the results. [Louis, 1836; Lilienfeld and Lilienfeld, 1980]

Louis's use of the word *indiscriminately* led Lilienfeld and Lilienfeld to wonder whether he had the concept of randomization in mind. The italics were evidently added by those authors.

Eventually, the ideas and methods of Louis not only put an end to bloodletting but also prompted physicians to reconsider other established treatments and principles. Thus, by the middle of the 19th century, real progress had been made, and the door was opened for medicine to become truly scientific and to escape from myths, superstitions, and traditions that could not stand up to scrutiny. Physicians and their medical co-workers gradually came to be regarded as professionals entitled to respect. Even though statistical tabulations began to appear more often in medical papers, it would take almost another century for physicians, statisticians, and mathematicians to become more closely allied.

CHAPTER 2

Statistics Becomes
a Distinct Discipline

Francis Bisset Hawkins's *Elements of Medical Statistics* was the first book in English concerned solely with medical statistics. Printed in 1829, it is, according to Greenwood (1943), a slender volume that is similar in format and size to the *Principles of Medical Statistics* published a little more than a century later by Sir Austin Bradford Hill. Some of the methods still used today were described before 1829 and were reported by Hawkins.

> Hawkins defined three indices he used in medical statistics: the ordinary crude death-rate—always expressed as one death in such or such a number; the probable life, i.e., the age to which half those born attain; and the mean life, i.e., the average age at death. [Greenwood, 1943]

Hawkins was aware that the age and sex constitution of a group affects the death rate. He wrote:

> In discussing the mortality of manufacturing towns or districts, it is just to remark that the small proportion is not always real; because a constant influx of adults is likely to render the number of deaths less considerable than that which could occur in a stationary population composed of all ages. [Greenwood, 1943]

"Hawkins was instrumental in obtaining the insertion of a column for the names of diseases or other causes of death, in connection with the first Act for the registration of births and deaths" (*Morton's Medical Bibliography*, 1991).

What Are Figures Worth?

John Snow (1813–1858)

From its earliest beginnings, medical statistics has been concerned with epidemics. An early illustration of the practical advantage of using the statistical method when confronted with a single specific disease in a limited geographical area was John Snow's study of the cause-and-effect association between the water supply of London and the spread of cholera (Underwood, 1951). In 1848, Snow began investigating the source and propagation of cholera. He and other physicians believed that the poison of cholera was taken directly into the alimentary canal through the mouth because the early symptoms were usually severe diarrhea and vomiting. The water supply became a primary suspect. Snow published his views in a pamphlet, *The Mode of Communication of Cholera*, in 1849.

During the cholera epidemics of 1832 and 1849, unusually high mortality occurred in districts supplied water by the Southwark and Vauxhall and the Lambeth companies. Both firms drew their water from the Thames River, which also received London's sewage. In 1853, however, the Lambeth Company moved "from central London to Thames Ditton, where the river was wholly free from the sewage of the metropolis" (Hill, 1953); the Southwark and Vauxhall Company continued as before.

The companies were competitors so that in some districts the pipes of each went along all of the streets and alleys. Snow (1855) noted:

> Each company supplies both rich and poor, both large houses and small. . . . No fewer than 300,000 people of both sexes, of every age and occupation, and of every rank and station, from gentlefolk down to the very poor, were divided into two groups without their choice, and, in most cases, without their knowledge; one group being supplied with water containing the sewage of London, and, amongst it, whatever might have come from the cholera patients, the other group having water quite free from such impurity. [Hill, 1953]

During the great epidemic in London in 1854, Snow and his assistant systematically investigated and recorded each death. They went up and down the streets listing for each household, the age and sex of all residents, the address, and the name of the company that

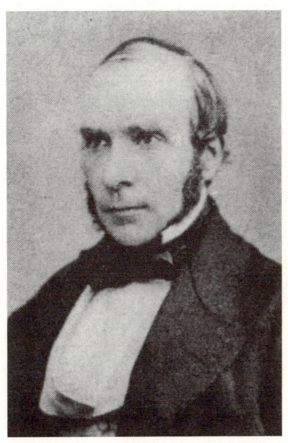

John Snow.

supplied their water. With persistent and accurate fieldwork they gathered the data necessary to explain the vital statistics.

In 40,000 houses served by Southwark and Vauxhall, 286 fatal attacks were found in the first 4 weeks of the epidemic—71 deaths per 10,000 households; in 26,000 houses served by the Lambeth Company, 14 fatal attacks were found—only 5 deaths per 10,000 households (Snow, 1855; Hill, 1953). The former company supplied water containing fecal sewage, while the Lambeth water was pure.

In one instance, a particularly virulent outbreak of cholera occurred in the neighborhood of Broad Street, Golden Square. About 500 fatalities were recorded in 10 days. The residents panicked and fled the city, but Dr. Snow intensified his research. He fixed his attention on the Broad Street pump as the source of the calamity and advised removal of the pump handle. Once the citizens were deprived of this water source and were advised to observe measures of extreme cleanliness when caring for patients, the epidemic ceased (Richardson, 1887). Snow later proved that the water from the Broad Street well was contaminated (Lord, 1889; Hill, 1953).

After reviewing Snow's account, however, Bradford Hill (1953) pointed out that the cholera outbreak had been declining for 5 or 6 days before the pump was inactivated. The reduction in cholera cases may have been related also to the escape from London of a sizable portion of the population and to the natural ebb of the epidemic.

In 1855, an expanded edition of Snow's original pamphlet was published as a book that contained all of his painstaking documentation as well as maps showing the origin and spread of the outbreaks.

Snow's report is "an epidemiological masterpiece, in which he showed conclusively that cholera is a transmissible disease that can be spread by water as well as by contact" (Ingraham, 1958). Wade Hampton Frost commented that Snow's book should be read once as a story of exploration and many times as a lesson in epidemiology. Hill added that the first time it should be read quickly, for its fascination, and then, like all closely-reasoned statistical studies, it must be taken slowly, carefully, and critically, with every piece of evidence weighed by the reader and its relevance studied (Frost, 1965; Hill, 1955).

Snow had neither the benefit of laboratory help nor knowledge of bacteriology or virology, but his work led to the eventual "purification of water supplies with the consequent saving of human lives from cholera, typhoid fever, dysentery, and other minor water-borne plagues" (Ingraham, 1958).

In 1937, an editor of the *British Medical Journal* stated that William

Farr later adopted Snow's method of investigation and, in a report of an epidemic in 1866, Farr reported:

> Many of the people [supplied by Southwark and Vauxhall] were in the habit of tying a piece of linen or some other fabric over the tap by which the water entered the butt or cistern, and in two hours, as the water came in, about a tablespoon of dirt was collected, all in motion with a variety of water insects, while the strained water was far from clear. [*Br Med J* 2:595–96, 1937]

William Farr (1807–1883)

After the age of 2 years, William Farr was cared for by an elderly benefactor who subsequently left a legacy to cover the completion of Farr's formal studies. Farr practiced and taught medicine and, to supplement his income, wrote, mainly about vital statistics, for medical journals, including a long series for *Lancet*, in 1835–36.

After he was appointed to the General Register Office (GRO) in 1839, he left his practice and devoted the next 40 years to creating and developing a national system of vital statistics that "not only popularised sanitary questions in England in such a manner as to render rapid health progress an accomplished fact, but which has, practically, been adopted in all the civilized countries of the world" (Farr, 1885, p. xiii).

Farr's writings on vital statistics encompassed many topics: population; marriages; births; deaths; life tables; sickness and health insurance; elementary education; civil registration of marriages, births, and deaths; present and future economic value of man; risk of fatal railway accidents; insurance against death or injury through railway accidents; and family nomenclature in England and Wales with most common surnames (Farr, 1885). His *Vital Statistics, or the Statistics of Health, Sickness, Disease and Death* appeared in McCulloch's *Statistical Account of the British Empire* in London in 1837. Greenwood ranks this publication only slightly below John Graunt's *Observations* as an original contribution to medical/statistical science (Greenwood, 1943). According to Greenwood, Farr used the methods of his predecessors and did not comment on defects of the data. He called attention to particular rates of mortality, for instance, those in the military:

> The soldier, in the prime of his physical powers, is rendered more liable to death every step he takes from his native climate, till at last the man of 28 years is subject, in the West Indies, to the same

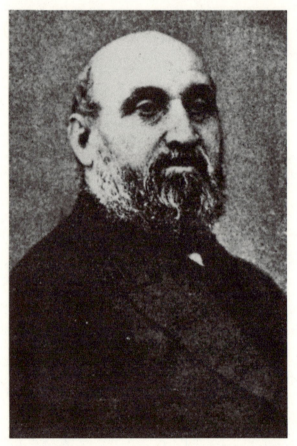

William Farr. (From *Vital Statistics: Memorial Volume of Selections from the Reports and Writings of William Farr*, 1975. The photograph is from a negative by Lombardi, Pall Mall. Courtesy of the New York Academy of Medicine.)

mortality as the man of 80 remaining in Britain. [Farr, 1837; Greenwood, 1943]

According to Farr's table, the average strength of British troops in Jamaica and Honduras between 1810 and 1828 was 2528 men. In the year of least mortality the death rate was 47 per 1000 men, with the average being 113 deaths and the maximum being 472! In the United Kingdom, the average death rate was 15 per 1000 people.

William Farr also wrote *English Life Table. Tables of Lifetimes, Annuities, and Premiums* (1864), for which he introduced the computer to medical statistics. "The appendix describes the use of the Scheutz version of Charles Babbage's calculating machine in the construction of the English Life Table No. 3. However, the machine required constant attention, and the GRO soon reverted to manual calculations employing logarithms until conversion to mechanical calculations in 1911" (*Morton's Medical Bibliography*, 1991, p. 265).

Farr lived to create the best official vital statistics system in the world (Greenwood, 1943). Diamond and Stone wrote:

> A highly competent government statistician, Farr was no outstanding mathematician, and his biographer, Eyler, notes the improvement in the quality of the mathematics of the statistical section of the British Association which followed his retirement and the election of Sir Francis Galton to replace him as President of the section. Farr's strength lay in an ability to glean from the paucity of statistical material available in nineteenth-century England the greatest possible practical information. [Diamond and Stone, 1981; Eyler, 1971]

Florence Nightingale (1820–1910)

This enterprising and energetic nurse had an early interest in hospital planning and operation that influenced her close attention to statistics. After making innovative changes in nursing care and in the management of some London hospitals, she advocated a uniform classification of all London hospital records and later was invited to reform two military hospitals in Scutari during the Crimean War in 1854. The hospitals were makeshift structures that were grimy, repulsive, and without adequate facilities to handle the medical or sanitary needs of the patients. Florence Nightingale and her corps of 38 nurses, working day and night, managed to establish routines of cleanliness

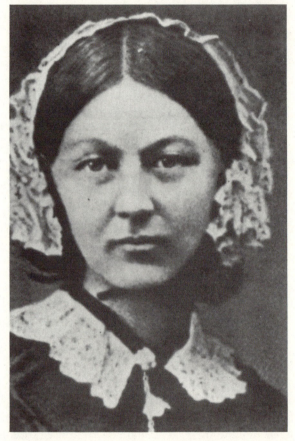

Florence Nightingale. (From Brown, P., 1989, *Florence Nightingale*, p. 5. Courtesy of George Weidenfeld & Nicolson, Ltd., London.)

and order and made radical changes that transformed the treatment of the common soldier. She was considered a national heroine in Britain.

After the Crimean War, the Prime Minister of Britain, Lord Palmerston, requested that she write about her experiences and comment on the necessary reforms; he was interested in establishing an Army Medical School and a Royal Commission (Cook, 1925). Nightingale especially wanted Farr on the new commission because he was a pioneer in the science of statistics, and she intended to compare the rates of sickness and death in barracks with those rates in civilian life. She believed the disparity would be shocking. The mortality of the Crimean disaster (73% in 6 months from diseases alone) was not caused by the war but by the system and bureaucracy that "controlled the health administration of the British Army" (Woodham-Smith, 1950). Nightingale's comprehensive suggestions for reforms became the 1000-page volume, *Notes of Matters Affecting the Health, Efficiency, and Hospital Administration of the British Army*, which was never published; she had a few copies privately printed (Woodham-Smith, 1950, p. 205).

During previous investigations, Nightingale had looked into the statistical records of London hospitals and realized that each institution went its own way. With the advice of Farr, she drafted a "standard classification of diseases and a set of model forms for Uniform Hospital Statistics" and wrote a paper for the International Statistical Congress, which met in London in 1860 (Nightingale, 1860; Cook, 1925, pp. 262–63). Nightingale did not present her report in person because she had become an invalid since her return from Crimea and in 1860 was confined to her home. She offered her house to Farr, however, so he could rest or bring delegates to dine and converse. One of the guests was Adolphe Quetelet, for whom she developed an admiration bordering on adulation (Diamond and Stone, 1981). Nightingale delighted in Quetelet's *Physique Sociale* and made many marginal annotations in her 1869 edition (now housed in the University College, London, library). She provided a copy of Quetelet's 1869 edition to Oxford University when she was urging officials to introduce statistics into the curriculum (Diamond and Stone, 1981).

In 1864, assisted by Farr, she prepared *Suggestions in regard to Sanitary Works required for the Improvement of Indian Stations*. She was concerned not only with the British soldiers but also with the Indian population, calling attention to conditions in civilian hospitals, jails, and "lunatic asylums," as well as the need for improvements in sanitation and hygiene in the towns (Cook, 1925, pp. 251–52). She wrote,

"Health is the product of civilisation, i.e., of real civilisation." After many of her suggestions had been carried out, the death rate from disease in the British army in India was far below the target figure (10 per 1000) set by the Royal Commission (Cook, 1925, pp. 251–52). Before her restorative projects, the average annual death rate for British soldiers in India had been 69 per 1000 (Cook, 1925, p. 245).

Although Nightingale had been educated at home and had received some tutoring in mathematics, she was a nurse and depended on Farr and others for information from official sources and for the statistical tables and diagrams used in her reports (Newell, 1984). It seems that neither Farr nor Nightingale had any interest in theoretical mathematics or abstract statistical principles but rather took a practical view of numbers. "What are figures worth—if they do no good to men's bodies or souls?" asked Farr (Diamond and Stone, 1981). Nightingale required statistical facts to bolster or reinforce her appeals for improvements in sanitation and in hospital administration. Cope (1958) reported that she apparently asked for information not to "ascertain truth of a doubtful question, but to enable her to be provided with arguments which she could use to support her already definitely held convictions."

Stunning Success

Louis Pasteur (1822–1895)

Louis Pasteur's extensive studies of germ theory and immunity established the background for his many successful trials. He had already investigated fermentation for the wine industry, had developed pasteurization, and was working on diseases of the silkworm when he sustained his first stroke at the young age of 46. He lived for an additional 27 productive years.

By the end of 1880, Pasteur had become proficient in the technique of artificially attenuating a virus and subsequently vaccinating with the weakened virus. In this way, he had created vaccines against fowl cholera, swine erysipelas, and anthrax. The vaccine of chicken cholera was not hard to acquire because pure cultures allowed to stand for a period of time in contact with air soon lost their virulence. The spores of anthrax, however, were not affected by air and retained a very prolonged virulence. After 8, 10, or 12 years, spores taken from the graves of victims of splenic fever (anthrax) were still in full virulent activity

(Vallery-Radot, 1923). Pasteur developed a process that acted on the bacilli before the spores were formed. He believed that his vaccine worked, and after performing laboratory tests on sheep, announced his success. There was much joking throughout France about his "cultivating microbes," and a public experiment was requested by the Melun Agricultural Society. Pasteur responded, "What has succeeded in the laboratory on fourteen sheep will succeed just as well at Melun on fifty" (Vallery-Radot, 1923). He had committed himself and had no retreat.

In 1881, under the glare of wide publicity, he carried out the experiment of his new vaccine against anthrax. Twenty-five sheep were given two inoculations (12 days apart) of the prophylactic vaccine. Fourteen days after the second vaccination, those 25 sheep and 25 unvaccinated sheep were injected with a virulent anthrax culture. Two days later Pasteur wrote to his children:

> It is only Thursday, and I am already writing to you; it is because a great result is now acquired. A wire . . . has just announced it. On Tuesday last, 31st May, we inoculated all the sheep, vaccinated and non-vaccinated, with very virulent splenic fever. It is not forty-eight hours ago. Well, the telegram tells me that, when we arrive at two o'clock this afternoon, all the non-vaccinated subjects will be dead; eighteen were already dead this morning, and the others dying. As to the vaccinated ones, they are all well; the telegram ends by the words "stunning success." [Vallery-Radot, 1923]

Pasteur suffered a second stroke at the age of 65; he continued to work but at a slower pace until he died at 73 of uremia and possibly another stroke (Mann, 1964).

Joseph Lister, First Baron (1827–1912)

In 1865, Joseph Lister was a surgeon at the Glasgow Royal Infirmary when he became acquainted with Pasteur's work on microorganisms; the same year he began using carbolic acid as an antiseptic in surgery.

Lister conducted small but extremely conclusive trials to confirm the effectiveness of antisepsis; these trials were described in *Lancet* (1870). Before Lister's program, pyemia, erysipelas, and gangrene were widespread among postsurgical patients, and he recorded the deaths in the male orthopedic surgery unit. Before his plan of action was introduced, 16 of 35 postsurgical patients died. During the 9 months after Lister instituted the use of antisepsis, only 6 of 40 postsurgical patients

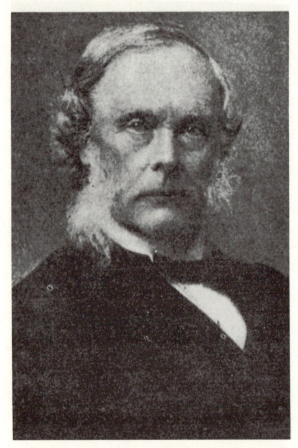

Lord Joseph Lister.

died, a reduction from 1 death in 2.2 persons to 1 in every 6.6. Lister (1870) wrote: "These numbers are, no doubt, too small for a satisfactory statistical comparison; but, when the details are considered, they are highly valuable with reference to the question we are considering." Bull (1959) commented that "the numbers are not at fault for the chi square test shows them to be highly significant; what is more open to question is the adequacy of the comparison with previous experience. . . ."

The effectiveness of Lister's antiseptic surgical procedures is best demonstrated by comparing his data for patients undergoing amputation of any part of an upper limb because there happened to be 12 such cases before he introduced antisepsis and 12 afterward. In the former group, 6 of 12 patients died, whereas only 1 of 12 patients died in the latter group (that patient died from pyemia despite surgery, not as a result of it, because he had suppuration of a metacarpal bone that continued after his hand was amputated). Although Lister's specific procedure is no longer used, his conviction that it is imperative to prevent microorganisms from gaining access to an operative incision continues to be a fundamental precept of modern surgery.

The Royal Statistical Society

Strangely, the motto chosen by the founders of the Statistical Society in 1834 was *Aliis exterendum*, which means "Let others thrash it out." William Cochran confessed that "it is a little embarrassing that statisticians started out by proclaiming what they will not do" (Cochran, 1976, 1982).

The original aims were given as "procuring, arranging, and publishing Facts calculated to illustrate the Conditions and Prospects of Society" (I. D. Hill, 1984), and the prime concern for the next 50 years seems to have been data collection. Hill wrote that practically nothing on mathematical methods or probability theory was published from 1834 to 1885. In one of the few publications that mentioned mathematics, *On the Relative Value of Averages Derived from Different Numbers of Observations*, the author concluded "that the formulae of the mathematician have a very limited application to the results of observation; and that if incautiously applied, they may lead to very grave errors" (Guy,1850; I. D. Hill, 1984).

In the 1885 Jubilee volume of the *Journal of the Statistical Society*, the first signs of a change of focus appeared. A paper by Francis Y. Edgeworth included probability, the normal curve, use of the median, parametric versus nonparametric tests, and the tendency of a mean toward normality (Edgeworth, 1885; I. D. Hill, 1984). Hill wrote that it was apparent from the discussion that few in the audience understood what Edgeworth was talking about. In the same issue, Galton introduced quartiles and percentiles (Galton, 1885). This renewed interest in mathematical statistics and Queen Victoria's 1887 grant of a royal charter that renamed the group the Royal Statistical Society (I. D. Hill, 1988) brought additional attention to statistics.

Statistics as a field was also advanced by the founding of the Societé de Statistique de Paris in 1803 and of the American Statistical Society in 1839. The first meeting of the International Statistical Congress was held in Brussels in 1853. After eight additional sessions, it was succeeded by the International Statistical Institute (ISI) in 1885 (Pollock, 1953).

Do You Wonder Where the k in Biometrika Comes From?

Francis Y. Edgeworth (1845–1926)

Francis Edgeworth was a true scholar who read and wrote in a number of languages, both ancient and modern. He seems to have been an individualist: he never married and his will "required the executors to destroy any manuscripts in his handwriting found in his rooms" (Kendall, 1970). Edgeworth was educated at Trinity College, Dublin, and at Oxford, but his background in mathematics is vague. He was very competent in algebra and calculus, which, possibly, he taught himself.

Edgeworth lectured in logic at King's College, London, where he became a professor of political economics and held a chair in economic science. He wrote *Mathematical Psychics* (1881) and advocated using mathematics to advance economic analysis. He also invented indifference curves and utility surfaces, which have become an accepted part of economic reasoning (Kendall, 1970). About this time in his career, he became interested in probability and, over the next 5 years, he published 25 articles on probability, least squares, index numbers, and variation in the value of money. In 1891, he was appointed to a chair in political economy at Oxford, and he became the first editor of the *Economic Journal*. Kendall (1970) summarized Edgeworth's contributions to statistics:

A good deal of Edgeworth's work in probability theory has been over-ridden by later writers and is of no special interest except as a record of the way in which the problems were considered at the time. Much of the same is true of his work on the best form of average and on correlation. There are three topics, however, to which he made lasting and important contributions. One is his work on index-numbers. The other two concern what nowadays would be called the theory of frequency distributions, but were then thought of as generalizations of the law of error.

Edgeworth admired Karl Pearson, and the two corresponded. Following Edgeworth's death in 1926, Pearson said that "like a good German, [Edgeworth] knew that the Greek *k* is not a modern *c*, and if any of you at any time wonder where the *k* in *Biometrika* comes from, I will frankly confess that I stole it from Edgeworth. Whenever you see that *k* call to mind dear old Edgeworth" (Kendall, 1970).

Some People Hate the Very Name of Statistics

Sir Francis Galton (1822–1911)

Sir Francis Galton's important statistical contributions were made gradually or piecemeal as he was trying to work out the principles of heredity. A half-cousin of Charles Darwin, Galton was interested in heredity and genetics, and "ordinary arithmetical methods were not sufficient for his purpose" (Underwood, 1951). Galton studied new ideas on the normal curve of error and relative values of averages derived from different numbers of observations, and then he developed these methods to a limited extent. His method of correlation, however, became his big contribution to statistics. In a paper published in 1888, he introduced the words *correlation* and *regression* in their technical sense (Galton, 1888; Underwood, 1951).

Galton, who had diverse interests in many fields of study, was perplexed by the narrow outlook of some statisticians of his day:

> It is difficult to understand why statisticians commonly limit their inquiries to Averages, and do not revel in more comprehensive views. Their souls seem as dull to the charm of variety as that of the native of one of our flat English counties, whose retrospect of Switzerland was that, if its mountains could be thrown into its lakes, two nuisances would be got rid of at once. . . .

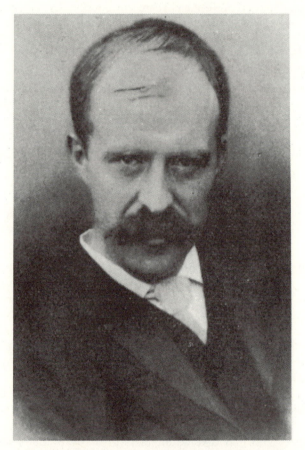

Walter Frank Raphael Weldon. (From Froggatt, P., and Nevin, N. C., 1971, The "law of ancestral heredity" and the Mendelian–ancestrian controversy in England 1889–1906. *J Med Genet* **8**:3. Courtesy of the British Medical Association and Mrs. E. J. Snell, for and on behalf of *Biometrika* trustees.)

Some people hate the very name of statistics, but I find them full of beauty and interest. Whenever they are not brutalised, but delicately handled by the higher methods, and are warily interpreted, their power of dealing with complicated phenomena is extraordinary. They are the only tools by which an opening can be cut through the formidable thicket of difficulties that bar the path of those who pursue the Science of man. [Galton, 1889; Forrest, 1974]

In 1893, the *Journal of the Royal Statistical Society* included the bivariate normal distribution described by Edgeworth, the correlation coefficient ascribed to Galton, and an abstract of a paper by Karl Pearson (on the mathematics of evolution) that used the term *standard deviation* (I. D. Hill, 1984). The modern field of statistics was taking shape, and future statisticians were being stimulated. For instance, Galton's *Natural Inheritance* (1889) had a dynamic influence on W. F. R. Weldon, who, in turn, prompted Karl Pearson to begin statistical studies.

Walter Frank Raphael Weldon (1860–1906)

Walter Weldon's father accumulated moderate wealth from discoveries in industrial chemistry. Before his father's death in 1885, Weldon lost a sister, a brother, and his mother. Weldon's inheritance made him independent, but his emotional nature and belief that he might not live to finish his chosen work may have been partially responsible for his inordinate intensity and apparent sense of urgency. Although he married, he and his wife had no children, and she remained free to assist in his zoologic experiments (Froggatt and Nevin, 1971).

When Weldon read Galton's work on frequency distributions and correlation, he recognized at once the possibilities for analyzing problems in evolution. The frequency of deviations from a type could be described specifically, and organic associations could be measured. Weldon immediately applied Galton's methods to a series of numerous measurements on the common shrimp (Weldon, 1890; Froggatt and Nevin, 1971). This work eventually confirmed Galton's belief that many organic measurements are normally distributed and that the degree of correlation between two organs is approximately the same for each local race of the species, with the regressions being linear (Weldon, 1892; Froggatt and Nevin, 1971). At this time, Weldon did not know Karl Pearson, whose son Egon S. Pearson wrote (1965) that Weldon's article of 1890 was almost certainly the first paper in which statistical methods were applied to biologic types other than man.

Early in 1891, Weldon was appointed to the Jodrell Chair in Zoology at University College, London, and in the summer of that year and at Easter 1892, he and his wife studied the Plymouth Sound shore crab and the Naples race of the same species. They measured 11 parameters of 2000 crab shells, and in only one instance was the distribution skewed. The curve was bimodal—*double-humped* was Weldon's term—and he showed that it could be a composite of two normal distributions (Froggatt and Nevin, 1971).

In late 1892, Weldon showed his curve and all his numbers to Karl Pearson in an appeal for mathematical guidance. Pearson tackled the subject head-on. He agreed with Weldon's logic of two normal populations compounding the double-humped curve, redid the statistical computations for Weldon's article, and for the first time, treated the dissection of a distribution assumed to be a composite of two or more normal distributions (K. Pearson, 1894; Froggatt and Nevin, 1971).

Weldon was a truly exacting researcher. Once when conducting experiments on dice-throwing, he rolled 12 dice 12,288 times, recording at each throw the number of dice showing more than 3 dots. (None may show more than 3 dots, or any number up to the whole 12—giving 13 possible results.) After a few tosses, he discovered that while there was no sign of regularity among the results, as the number of tosses increased, the frequency with which each of the 13 possible results occurred approached a constant and predictable percentage of the whole number. Likewise, in describing any characteristic of living things, he noted that "we are unable to predict the result of any single observation before we have made it, but we can predict, with very considerable accuracy, the result of a long series" (Weldon, 1906).

Would It Be Too Hopelessly Expensive to Start a Journal?

Karl Pearson (1857–1936)

Like Galton, Karl Pearson was a man of great intellect and many varied interests. In 1885, at age 28, he was appointed to the Chair of Applied Mathematics at University College, London. He had written on history, ethics, philosophy, art, and politics but very little on mathematics. *Natural Inheritance* stimulated his interest in heredity and evolution,

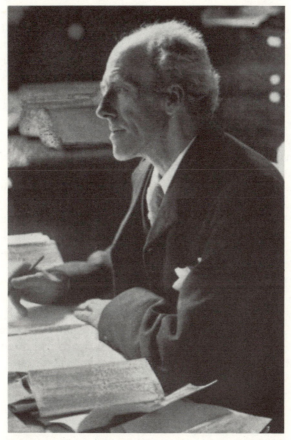

Karl Pearson. (From Pearson, E.S., 1937, Karl Pearson: An appreciation of some aspects of his life and work. *Biometrika* **29:**161. Courtesy of the British Medical Association and Mrs. E. J. Snell, for and on behalf of *Biometrika* trustees.)

but the catalyst was "Weldon's enthusiasm and vigor, his eagerness to have Darwinian evolution demonstrated by statistical inquiry" (Froggatt and Nevin, 1971). Pearson's long-standing relationships with Galton and Weldon were enduring stimuli to his creative output.

The year 1893 marked a turning point in Pearson's career—he found his professional mission. While developing procedures to help Weldon, Pearson "had ideas that required an advanced theory of statistics and this he founded in several series of papers" (Froggatt and Nevin, 1971). These articles became the foundation of modern mathematical statistics. In an astonishing profusion of publications, Pearson presented the "apparatus of moments and correlation, the system of frequency curves, the probable errors of moments and product-moments reached by maximizing the likelihood function, and the chi-square goodness-of-fit test, all in the space of 15 years when he was also lecturing many hours a week" (David, 1985). The term *standard deviation* was introduced by him in a lecture to the Royal Society in 1893. Pearson's work was the end result of background ideas from the previous two centuries (Hart, 1988).

In 1900, his first paper on the chi-square test for significance was published, and although it has undergone changes, it has had a considerable influence in all uses of statistical methods (Underwood, 1951). Cochran (1982, p. 49.316) wrote that the style of that paper had always impressed him as "unusual for a pioneering paper" because "Pearson wrote with the air of a man who knows exactly what he is doing. The exposition, although clear, is slightly hurried and brusque, as if the reader will not wish to be troubled by elaborate details of a problem that is routine and straight forward." Although Pearson created the chi-square test for goodness-of-fit to accommodate comparisons of observed and theoretical frequency curves, Weldon's double-humped curve enticed him to think about and examine the general theory of frequency curves (Froggatt and Nevin, 1971). Weldon believed that "recognizable mutations only contributed to evolution in exceptional circumstances and that evolution and selection were mass phenomena to be studied by statistical methods" (Froggatt and Nevin, 1971). That opinion and also the concept of *ancestral inheritance* put forth by Pearson and Weldon were "not received kindly by many biologists," and controversies ensued (David, 1985). William Bateson, a geneticist, was a particularly acrimonious critic.

Quarrels arose from prepublication reviews of submitted papers, and in 1900 the Royal Society rejected an important paper by Pearson, who firmly believed that "most biological work on statistical lines would suffer a similar fate in the future" (Pearson to Galton, 13 December 1900, in Forrest, 1974, pp. 251–52; K. Pearson, 1930).

In November 1900, Weldon wrote to Pearson: "The contention 'that numbers mean nothing and do not exist in Nature' will have to be fought. . . . Do you think it would be too hopelessly expensive to start a journal of some kind?" (Froggatt and Nevin, 1971). Pearson was enthusiastic, Galton gave 200 pounds to help launch the project, and *Biometrika: A Journal for the Statistical Study of Biological Problems* was born. Edited by Weldon, Pearson, and C. B. Davenport (an American) in consultation with Galton, volume one appeared in 1901.

In a short introduction to biometry, Galton explained that the journal was intended for those interested in the application of the modern methods of statistics to biology:

> The new methods occupy an altogether higher plane than that in which ordinary statistics and simple averages move and have their being. Unfortunately the ideas of which they treat, and still more the many technical phrases employed in them, are as yet unfamiliar. The arithmetic they require is laborious, and the mathematical investigations on which the arithmetic rests are difficult reading even for experts . . . this new departure in science makes its appearance under conditions that are unfavourable to its speedy recognition, and those who labour in it must abide for some time in patience before they can receive much sympathy from the outside world. [Galton, 1901]

The journal prospered, and Pearson and his students had a vehicle for publication of their important efforts. Later, it lost its biologic applications and became a preeminent outlet for statistical theory (Forrest, 1974, p. 252). Pearson edited the journal until his death in 1936.

Egon Pearson later wrote that in 1904, at the Cambridge meeting of the British Association for the Advancement of Science, William Bateson had entered the lecture hall carrying a parcel containing all of the back issues of *Biometrika* and had thrown them down on a table with the remark, "I hold that the whole of that is worthless." Weldon, sitting beside Pearson, muttered, "At least, we have got his subscription." But no, Bateson had brought the journals from the library of the Cambridge Philosophical Society (E.S. Pearson, 1970).

Galton advised that *Biometrika* should have "glossaries appended to papers in which there would appear biological terms such as *chromosome* and *zygote* to encourage the statisticians to read the articles, and that the mathematics of statistical papers should be simplified to aid their comprehension by the biologists" (Galton to Pearson, 8 March 1908, in Forrest, 1974, p. 277; K. Pearson, 1930, p. 334).

The conflict and contention with his peers affected Pearson, and he stopped participating in meetings of the scientific societies; he was never a fellow of the Royal Statistical Society (David, 1985; personal communication from the Royal Statistical Society, April, 1992). Weldon moved to a chair at Oxford in 1899, and Pearson became more isolated; his contacts with Weldon related primarily to editing *Biometrika*. Weldon died in 1906 from pneumonia at age 46. His widow later endowed a chair of biometry at University College, and in 1937, J. B. S. Haldane became its first occupant (Froggatt and Nevin, 1971).

> To Pearson, the loss of Weldon was irreparable and left "almost desolation": "how mentally refreshing it was to me being near him for a few weeks and how it sent me back fit for work with new vigor and new ideas. He always gave me courage and hope to go on . . . I seem now quite dazed . . . wholly without energy to start the term." [Froggatt and Nevin, 1971]

Forrest relates that Pearson leaned on Galton for sympathy and advice. A month after Weldon's death, Pearson felt he could no longer continue the struggle to have biometric work published outside his own *Biometrika*. The Royal Society [not to be confused with the Royal Statistical Society] had again rejected a paper, and in despair Pearson wrote to Galton to ask whether he should resign his fellowship (Pearson to Galton, 13 May 1906, in Forrest, 1974, p. 268; K. Pearson, 1930, p. 282). Galton's reply was a model of sound advice.

> Dear Karl Pearson, I fully understand and sympathise with your feelings. It is a disgrace to the biologists of the day, that their representatives in the Royal Society are incapable of understanding biometric papers, and of distinguishing between bad and good statistical work. To that extent I am entirely at one with you, but I do not on the above grounds see that your resignation would mend matters. It is a very general rule of conduct not to withdraw when in a minority, because a vantage ground is surrendered by doing so. It is far easier to reform a society while a member of it than when an outsider. . . . So I should say don't resign, but abide your time, and give a good and well-deserved slash now and then to serve as a reminder that your views are strong, though not querulously and wearisomely repeated. [Galton to Pearson, 14 May 1906, in Forrest, 1974, p. 268; K. Pearson, 1930, p. 283]

Galton was 67 years old when *Natural Inheritance* was published, and he filled the role of a mentor to Pearson. Forrest (1974, p. 193) tells us that "Pearson was well aware of several mathematic fallacies in Galton's work and, out of respect and admiration for the man, introduced 'enormous complexities' in his own attempts to verify Galton's statements." "Some of Galton's regression values were incorrect and the data was reworked by Pearson" (Forrest, 1974, pp. 203–04). Galton helped to fund a biometrics laboratory, and when he died in 1911, money was left for a chair in eugenics, which Pearson was the first to occupy. The biometrics laboratory and Galton's eugenics laboratory both became part of the new Department of Applied Statistics at University College, London, with Pearson in charge as the Galton Professor (David, 1985; Peters, 1987, p. 106). Years earlier Florence Nightingale had asked Galton to aid her in creating such a professorship for the statistical study of social problems—issues in education, criminology, etc. (H. L. Walker, 1929; Peters, 1987, p. 106).

Pearson wrote *Life, Letters and Labours of Francis Galton*, a three-volume tribute completed in 1930, as a memorial to his friend.

> Again, if the reader anticipates that Galton was a faultless genius, who solved his problems straight away without slip or doubtful procedure, he is bound to be disappointed. Some creative minds may have done that, or appear to have done it, because, the building erected, they left no signs of the scaffolding; but the majority of able men stumble and grope in the twilight like their lesser brethren, only they have the persistency and insight which carries them on to the dawn. [K. Pearson, 1930, p. 6]

After 1900, teaching flourished for Karl Pearson. His lectures attracted students and professors from all parts of the world who then went home to apply Pearson's mathematical principles and to teach others. During the years of World War I, there was "great uncertainty about the future of *Biometrika*." In a letter to R. A. Fisher, Pearson wrote that the war had cut off the bulk of the continental subscribers and that Cambridge Press had declined to give aid (Pearson to Fisher, 13 May 1916, in Box 1978*). Pearson alone was responsible for the journal. His staff was depleted, he was doing war work, and the publication of

---

*All citations in this book credited to Box (1978) refer to Joan Fisher Box: *R. A. Fisher: The Life of a Scientist*. New York: John Wiley & Sons, Inc. Reprinted by permission of John Wiley & Sons, Inc.

papers was often delayed. The years after World War I, identified by many as the period of bitter contention between Pearson and Fisher, are more significant historically for the promotion of statistics to a proper position in university curricula and for the widespread teaching of how to analyze data (David, 1985).

Egon Pearson wrote that his father was very interested in historical studies, and after reading a series of Karl's lectures on the mathematics of statistics in the medieval and renaissance periods, it is easy to understand why he attracted large audiences. These were given at University College, London, between 1921 and 1933. For example:

> We find him giving a picture of John Graunt against the background of the London of Charles II; the Great Plague and the early meetings of the Royal Society and of Sir William Petty's profitable ventures in Ireland. A little later we find him clearly fascinated by the life and character of Edmund Halley; besides a description of his famous Life Table we have therefore an account of Halley's astronomical interests, his stay in St. Helena to locate the stars of the southern hemisphere and his later Atlantic cruises from northern to southern icefields as Captain of *H. M. S. Paramour*, seeking by observation the causes of the variation of the compass. [K. Pearson, 1978, preface]

Karl Pearson also emphasized the extent to which "the bright promise of the 'scientific Renaissance' was held in check by the stubborn belief in biblical theory . . ." (K. Pearson, 1978, preface). The compilation of his lectures, *The History of Statistics in the 17th and 18th Centuries Against the Changing Background of Intellectual, Scientific and Religious Thought*, is captivating reading for anyone interested in statistics, mathematics, or history.

Karl Pearson retired in 1933. His department was divided into the Department of Eugenics, with Fisher as the Galton Professor, and the Department of Statistics under Egon Pearson, who was responsible for undergraduate teaching. Karl Pearson died in 1936, and Helen L. Walker (1958) wrote:

> What he did in moving the scientific world from a state of sheer disinterest in statistical studies over to a situation in which a large number of well trained persons were eagerly at work developing new theory, gathering and analyzing statistical data from every content field, computing new tables, and reexamining the foundations of statistical philosophy, is an achievement of fantastic proportions. . . . Few men in all the history of science have stimulated so

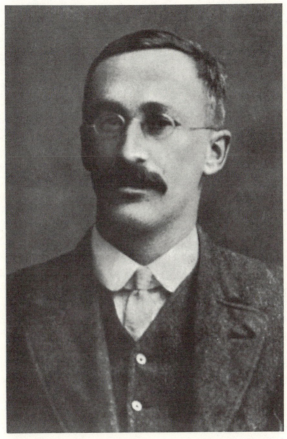

William S. Gosset ("Student"). (From Fisher, R.A., 1939, "Student." *Ann Eugen* **9**:1. Courtesy of Cambridge University Press.)

many other people to cultivate and enlarge the fields they had planted.

Following Karl Pearson's death, his son edited *Biometrika* from 1936 to 1966, and he was succeeded by Sir David R. Cox from January 1966 through December 1990, prompting the Chairman of the Trustees (Peter Armitage) to remark, "The Trustees are unlikely to be able to guarantee the continuation of the arithmetic progression so far established (in their choice of a new editor)" (Armitage, 1990). Karl Pearson had served for 35 years, Egon Pearson for 30 years, and David Cox for 25 years. Over the years, the emphasis of the articles in *Biometrika* has shifted in response to changing needs, and now it is widely regarded as the world's leading journal for general statistical methodology.

Two Hours of Hard Work

William Sealy Gosset ("Student") (1876–1937)

After obtaining a degree in chemistry and mathematics at Oxford, William Gosset worked for the Guinness brewery in Dublin, Ireland. While investigating the variations in the quality of barley and hops from different sources, circumstances of preparation, and the finished yield, he became interested in describing exact error probabilities of statistics from small samples (Read, 1983).

Before Gosset's time, when statisticians did not know the standard deviations of the populations they were studying, they relied on large samples for which the estimates of the standard deviations were presumed to be close to their true values. For example, Peters (1987, pp. 108–09) noted that George Yule (1911) used an 1883 report that had listed the heights of 8585 males in Great Britain; Yule's discussion included data published by K. Pearson and Lee in 1903 on the heights of 1078 father and son pairs. Gosset realized that his sample sizes would be small, and he was unsure about analyzing his data. He consulted Karl Pearson in 1905 (Peters, 1987, p. 109), and, subsequently, his employers arranged for Gosset to spend a year (1906–07) studying under Pearson (Read, 1983).

Gosset took his small-sample problem along to London, and after learning the theory of correlation and the Pearson system of frequency curves, began creating statistical skills to analyze small-sample data (Read, 1983). As Fisher later commented, "Little experience is sufficient to show that the traditional machinery of statistical processes is wholly unsuited to the needs of practical research. Not only does it take a cannon to shoot a sparrow, but it misses the sparrow!" (Fisher, 1925, preface; Box, 1978, p. 130).

Student's well-known paper, *The Probable Error of a Mean* (1908), was the first major step in attempting to quantify results of experimentation (Cochran, 1976).

> "Student" showed, in the particular case he treated, that it was possible to find a quantity, which was known to them as "Student's *t*," having a frequency distribution independent of all unknown parameters, and being at the same time expressible as a function of one only of these parameters, together with other quantities directly observable, and, therefore, known with exactitude. [Fisher, 1934]

Surprisingly, Gosset's "tables of percent points of the *t*-distributions were used by few researchers other than those at Guinness and Rothamsted [see Chapter 3] until the late 1920s" (Read, 1983). Fisher alone followed Gosset's lead in investigating sampling statistics, and, as shown by their correspondence, the two men collaborated from 1923 to 1925 in assembling these tables. By then, Fisher's work on the analysis of variance method for the comparison of two or more means was already requiring the reformulation of Student's test in terms of the now familiar Student's *t*. Snedecor (1937) later named the *F* test in honor of Fisher (Mainland, 1954).

> The use of "Student's " distribution enables us to appreciate the value of observing a sufficient number of parallel cases; their value lies, not only in the fact that the standard error of a mean decreases inversely as the square root of the number of parallels, but in the fact that the accuracy of our estimate of the standard error increases simultaneously. [Fisher (1925), 13th ed. 1958, p. 126]

At times, Gosset had difficulty following Fisher's reasoning and logic.

> It's not so much the mathematics, I can often say "Well, of course, that's beyond me, but we'll take it as correct" but when I come to 'Evidently' I know that it means two hours hard work at least before I can see why. [Gosset, 1970, no. 6; Box, 1981]

Gosset was dubious about using randomization for field experiments, and, "on this subject, Fisher never wholly convinced him" (Box,

1981). Before World War I, Gosset's work at the brewery led him to design the half-drill strip layout for comparing barley varieties. In 1936 he spoke (before the Royal Statistical Society) in favor of this design, which continued to be used for barley trials all over Ireland. Randomization had been introduced in the interval, but he preferred his balanced design over Fisher's randomized ones, claiming that "since the tendency of deliberate randomising is to increase the error, balanced arrangement like the half-drill is best" (Student, 1936, 1937; Box, 1981). Gosset maintained that a systematic design was inherently more accurate than a randomized one (Box, 1981).

The correspondence between Gosset and Fisher reveals a growing friendship but also shows a continuing difference of opinion on this point. When Gosset made his public statement, Fisher openly opposed him, defending randomization. A heated debate followed, and Gosset's death in 1937 removed any chance for them to settle their conflict.

Gosset is remembered for introducing and developing problems related to small-sample distributions, which have occupied statisticians for many years. In a memorial article, Fisher wrote that Student, in his paper of 1908, had presented a fundamentally new approach to the problem of the theory of errors.

> "Student's" work has shown that a better course is open to us than that of adapting even the best available estimate of the variance of the population; that, by finding the exact sampling distribution of such an estimate, we may make allowance for its sampling errors, so as to obtain a test of significance which, in spite of these errors, is exact and rigorous. He thus rendered obsolete the restriction that the sample must be "sufficiently large." . . .
>
> It is doubtful if "Student" ever realized the full importance of his contribution to the Theory of Errors. . . . Probably he felt that, had the problem really been so important as it had once seemed, the leading authorities in English statistics would at least have given him the encouragement of recommending the use of his method; and, better still, would have sought to gain similar advantages in more complex problems. . . .
>
> It would not be too much to ascribe this to the increasing dissociation of theoretical statistics from the practical problems of scientific research. [Fisher, 1939]

Why did Gosset use the pseudonym Student? The Guinness Company had given permission for the publication of the first scientific paper by one of their employees on the condition that a pseudonym be used, possibly because competing companies might otherwise have become aware of the ongoing Guinness research (Box, personal communication, June, 1992; Reid, 1982, p. 54).

Idealism Recedes

By 1920, Karl Pearson was 63 years old, and the creative output and vigor of his younger years had waned. He continued to be a very capable editor of *Biometrika* and pursued his long-established interest in history. His son tells us that

> The post-war years were not favourable to the spread of Galton's eugenic creed. Too much idealism had been poured out vainly in the battlefields of France. [Pearson was not eager to return] to the task of urging man on to the improvement of his breed. [E. Pearson, 1937]

Use of the statistical method, however, was becoming more and more customary and accepted. A growing number of students at University College were working toward honors degrees in statistics, which had been instituted a few years earlier. Lecturing and assisting undergraduates occupied a large segment of Pearson's time and energy.

With talent, expertise, and hard work, Karl Pearson earned his reputation as the predominant figure of his time in multiple areas—statistics, biometry, evolution, and eugenics. As is often the case, when an acknowledged leader in any occupation begins to ease up, a younger, fresh, dynamic person assumes center stage—and that is exactly what happened in the field of statistics.

CHAPTER 3

Researchers and Statisticians Come Together

Before the 1920s clinical physicians, researchers, mathematicians, and statisticians had separate, somewhat segregated, spheres of work that were usually unrelated. These professionals did not ordinarily come together to attack problems, but between 1920 and 1950 a change gradually occurred.

> the growing use of quantitative methods in medicine may be regarded as a potent factor, and in turn as an important result, of the recent and most welcome weakening of the attitude of critical aloofness which formerly prevailed. . . . [Dale, 1951]

During this period, Sir Ronald Fisher was the acknowledged leader in developing statistical theory, and Sir Austin Bradford Hill was the forerunner in applying statistical principles in medicine.

Sir Ronald Aylmer Fisher (1890–1962)

Endowed with Talent

Joan Fisher Box wrote a very sensitive and comprehensive biography, *R. A. Fisher: The Life of a Scientist*, that provides a more extended version of his life and work than given here.

Ronald Fisher was a surviving twin (Gridgeman, 1971), and his mathematical aptitude was apparent at an early age. When he was

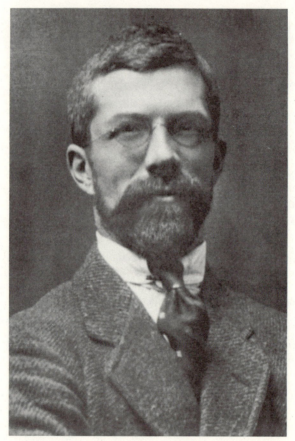

Sir Ronald Aylmer Fisher in 1924. (From Box, J. F., 1978, *R. A. Fisher: The Life of a Scientist*, plate 4. Copyright © 1978, John Wiley & Sons, Inc. By permission of John Wiley & Sons, Inc.)

about 3 years old, he asked one morning, "What is a half of a half?" After his nurse answered that it was a quarter, there was a pause before he asked, "And what is a half of a quarter?" She told him that it was an eighth, and there was a longer pause before he asked again, "What is half of an eighth?" After she responded, there was a long silence until, finally, the tiny child said slowly, "Then, I suppose that a half of a sixteenth must be a thirty-toof" (Box, 1978, pp. 12–13).

Extremely limited vision was an inconvenience throughout Fisher's life; in 1904 he dropped out of school for a term to rest his eyes. His mother read aloud to him until her death (also in 1904) from acute peritonitis, following which his sisters and wife, in turn, assumed this responsibility. His tutorials in mathematics at Harrow were accomplished without pencil and paper or any visual aid. Later, he dictated nonmathematical papers to a great extent; his wife literally took down all but two chapters of *The Genetical Theory of Natural Selection* word for word at his dictation (Box, 1978, p. 186).

Fisher's excellence in mathematics won him scholarships at the age of 14 to Harrow and at age 19 to Cambridge as an undergraduate in mathematics and later as a postgraduate student of the theory of errors, statistical mechanics, and quantum theory (Box, 1983).

A Focus on Eugenics

While Fisher was at Cambridge (1909–1913), the science of genetics was granted academic recognition, and the Balfour Chair of Genetics was permanently endowed in 1912 (Box, 1978, p. 22). Fisher was exposed to lively discussions, not only of genetics but also of evolution and natural selection, and, of prime interest to him, eugenics. In 1911, he promoted the creation of the Cambridge University Eugenics Society, whose members desired to educate themselves and conduct research in eugenics. Fisher led the undergraduate activities of the group, served on the council, and was the principal speaker at the society's second annual meeting in 1912.

Leaving Cambridge at the age of 23, he joined the Eugenics Education Society of London, which he served until 1934. He became a regular reviewer for the *Eugenics Review*, evaluating more than 200 books; during the 1920s, he did all of the reviewing of statistical and genetical work. His early interest in eugenics continued throughout his life as revealed by his numerous publications.

Early Frustrations

In London, Fisher began working as a statistician for the Mercantile and General Investment Company. He considered the job temporary, expecting military recruitment. When he volunteered for active duty in 1914, however, the army rejected him because of his eyesight. Bitterly disappointed, he tried repeatedly to enter the service. His brother was on duty in France, his sister worked in an emergency hospital in England, and most of his friends had enlisted in combat units (Box, 1978, p. 36).

Being excluded from military service, Fisher served his country for the next 5 years by teaching physics and mathematics in several boys' schools. He hated teaching, and his inability to transmit his own enthusiasm for learning to the young students plus his experiences with other teachers led to his developing a low opinion of the profession. Later, he never once visited the schools attended by any of his eight children (Box, 1978, pp. 36–37). Fisher found himself in a boring, unfulfilling situation and began to consider farming as a man's life and as a means of helping to solve the wartime food shortages. Thus, when he began teaching at Bradfield College, Berkshire, in 1917, he rented a former gamekeeper's cottage on the Bradfield estate to have land available to gain experience in subsistence farming and animal husbandry.

The same year, Fisher married; a son, George, was born in 1919 and a daughter, Katie, in 1922. Katie died tragically when she was 5 months old, but, eventually, another son and six daughters were added to the family. The children were, perhaps, "a personal expression of his genetic and evolutionary convictions" (Gridgeman, 1971).

Publications (1912–1922)

As narrated in Chapter 2, Galton, Weldon, and Karl Pearson were all pioneers in applying statistical methods to the analysis of biologic data, but they were so strongly opposed by some biologists in the Royal Society that they finally felt compelled to create their own journal. In Fisher's very first paper to the undergraduate committee of the Cambridge University Genetics Society he used quantitative ideas to show that researchers in both genetics and biometry must contribute to advance the knowledge of human heredity.

In 1912, his first paper, *On an Absolute Criterion for Fitting Frequency Curves*, was published. In it, he introduced the method of maximum likelihood, although he did not name it "likelihood" until years later (Fisher, 1912; reprinted in Fisher 1971–74, paper 1).

"In 1915, Pearson published Fisher's article on the general sampling distribution of the correlation coefficient in *Biometrika* [Fisher, 1915] and went on to have the ordinates of the error of estimated correlations calculated in his department" (Box, 1983). Fisher was aware of this ongoing analysis and requested "copies of proofs of such of this work, as is complete" (Fisher to K. Pearson, 15 May 1916, Box, 1978, p. 78). There is no evidence that Fisher saw any proofs before the article by Soper *et al.* (1917) appeared in print. Thus, Fisher was shocked to find that the authors had criticized his work without contacting him before publication. "Pearson had not understood the method of maximum likelihood Fisher had used, and condemned it as being inverse inference, which Fisher had deliberately avoided" (Box, 1983). "What particularly upset Fisher . . . was the imputation that he had invoked Bayes' theorem with a uniform prior for p [probability of an event]; Pearson advocated an empirical prior which led to different numerical results" (Hinkley, 1980). This handling of Fisher's publication marked the beginning of a deep-seated ill will between him and Pearson.

"Fisher accepted Bayes' theorem and honored its orginator as the first to use the theory of probability as an instrument of inductive reasoning; however, from the beginning, he rejected Bayes' postulate" (Box, 1978, p. 449), listing three reasons for his position:

> (1) it leads to apparent mathematical contradictions, (2) the truth of an axiom should be apparent to any rational mind which fully comprehends its meaning, but Bayes' [postulate] does not carry this conviction of necessary truth, and (3) inverse probability has been only very rarely used in the justification of conclusions from experimental facts, although the theory has been widely taught. [Fisher, 1935]

Fisher used the Bayesian method only when prior probabilities were known (Box, 1978, p. 449).

Fisher continued to work on eugenics and inheritance, and, in 1916, *The Correlation to be Expected Between Relatives on the Supposition of Mendelian Inheritance* was submitted to the Royal Society. In this article, Fisher reconciled genetics and biometry. The referees were men of prestige in these two subjects: Karl Pearson, biometrician, and R. C. Punnett, geneticist. Pearson reported that "the paper was not of much interest from the biometric standpoint" and Punnett said that "whatever the paper's value from a biometric standpoint it was not of much interest to biologists" (Bennett, 1983). Thus, "it was too statistical for the one, too genetical for the other" (Box, 1978, p. 59). The paper (Fisher, 1918) was finally published 2 years later, with the publication cost being underwritten by the Eugenics Education Society and Leonard Darwin.

In 1919, Fisher received a letter from Karl Pearson.* This letter is reproduced here in its entirely as given in Bennett (1983, p. 117) because it clearly indicates that Fisher is invited merely to enter his name for consideration for a position at the Galton Laboratory and implies that he would have to forego his own interests in research and writing and concentrate on advancing Pearson's theories.

> Old Schoolhouse,
> Coldharbour,
> Near Dorking.
> August 2, 1919
>
> Dear Mr. Fisher,
>   Your name has been mentioned to me as a possible man for a post I have to fill at the Galton Laboratory, namely that of a senior assistant at 350 pounds per annum. I do not know whether the post would have inducements for you, and I fully realize that there would be difficulties in the way. I want a man who will throw himself wholeheartedly into the work at the Laboratory as it is at present organized, not a research worker who would follow his own individual lines regardless of the general scheme of work. A real taste for and patience in the somewhat laborious work of computing tabulating and reduction is essential. Mathematical knowledge is very essential, but it is in a sense secondary, i.e., we do not seek mathematical problems, we have quite enough as they arise in the ordinary course of our work. At the same time I, of course, endeavour to encourage all research tending to extend theory so far as it is of importance to our own subject. At the same time I like also primarily a man who has had experience of observations or measurements, and if possible has been through our special training in computing and statistics. I find as a rule that a high Cambridge wrangler [having a first-class honors degree in mathematics] usually takes two years to become an efficient practical statistician and computer, and that by this time or before he wants a more highly paid post than we can give. I want somebody

---

*Letter from Karl Pearson to R. A. Fisher, 1919. From Bennett, J. H., 1983, Darwin–Fisher correspondence 1915–1929. In *Natural Selection, Heredity, and Eugenics*, J. H. Bennett (ed.), p. 117. Courtesy of Oxford University Press.

who will stick loyally by the Laboratory for a number of years especially during the present critical time, when we are going into a new building with very considerable extension of our work and possibilities, but with inadequate funds owing to the war-conditions. I have one or two men in view, but as you have been specially mentioned from Cambridge I feel I must write to you among them and find out what your views may be. I may be in London for a day during August, if you cared for a talk, or this is not inaccessible via Reading and Dorking.

I am,

> Yours very sincerely,
> Karl Pearson

Fisher, instead, chose a temporary appointment as a statistician at Rothamsted Experimental Station.

Several years after its publication, Fisher responded to the article by Soper *et al.* (1917) by writing a paper in which he restated his concept of likelihood in a way that denied any dependence on Bayes's theorem. In addition, he presented a new z-transformation to reduce the skewed curves of the correlation coefficients to practically normal shape, for which the error distribution was easily available (Fisher, 1921). This z-transformation was valuable not only in the subsequent development of the analysis of variance but proved to be useful in other circumstances as well. Fisher used it to deal with a practical problem concerning the correlation between pairs of twins (Fisher, 1919) and to convert the curves for intraclass correlations to approximately normal. He included his derivation of the distribution of the intraclass correlation coefficient in a paper (Fisher, 1921) that he mailed to Pearson in 1920 (Box, 1978, pp. 80–83). Pearson replied:

> Only in passing through Town today did I find your communication of August 3rd. . . . As there has been a delay of three weeks already, and as I fear if I could give full attention to your paper, which I cannot at the present time, I should be unlikely to publish it in its present form, or without a reply to your criticisms which would involve also a criticism of your work of 1912—I would prefer you published elsewhere. Under present printing and financial conditions, I am regretfully compelled to exclude all that I think is erroneous on my own judgement, because I cannot afford controversy. [Box, 1978, p. 83]

Fisher vowed never again to submit a paper to Pearson's *Biometrika*, and he never did.

Another disagreement was aired in 1922 when the *Journal of the Royal Statistical Society* published Fisher's paper on the interpretation of chi-square and contingency tables. He named "degrees of freedom" on this occasion to clarify the idea. "For the 2 × 2 table Pearson's chi-square had been used with three degrees of freedom by Pearson, but Fisher's geometric insight led to the correct single degree of freedom" (Hinkley, 1980, p. 4). He showed that chi-square could be used in examples which, with Pearson's method, required special adjustment. The test was sometimes being used in research publications without regard for the special usage, and Fisher showed that this laxness could give erroneous results (Fisher, 1922a; Box, 1978, pp. 84–85).

Pearson responded harshly, arguing that dilemmas, doubts, and confusion existed in some areas with Fisher's approach. When Fisher attempted to explain, the editors of the *Journal of the Royal Statistical Society* declined publication—perhaps intimidated by the possibility of Pearson's wrath. Fisher eventually (1923) resigned from the Society (Box, 1978, pp. 86–87). Years later, Neyman (1976) wrote:

> The Pearson chi-square criterion for goodness-of-fit also necessitated the solution of a distribution problem. This was solved by Karl Pearson for the case in which the distribution supposed to fit the data is completely specified, involving no adjustable parameters. Originally, Pearson himself and his many followers thought that the presence of adjustable parameters to be estimated did not affect the distribution of chi-square.
>
> Using simulation sampling, G. Udny Yule became convinced to the contrary (Yule, 1922). Subsequently, in a series of investigations, beginning with one by R. A. Fisher (1924), it was established that the suspicions of Yule are justified—the distribution of chi-square was found to depend on the so-called number of degrees of freedom and on the method used to estimate the adjustable parameters.

In 1929, Fisher was reelected to the Royal Statistical Society in a peace-making gesture.

Work at Rothamsted

Six years after setting forth from Cambridge, Fisher was finally hired for a position in which he could apply his special skills. On receiving a temporary appointment at Rothamsted Experimental Station in 1919, Fisher assumed responsibility for "sorting and reassessing a sixty-six-year accumulation of data on manurial field trials and weather records" (Gridgeman, 1971).

One hundred and fifty years before Fisher began writing about crop studies, Arthur Young (1741–1820), another Englishman, had devoted his life to experiments designed to discover the most profitable methods of farming. He accomplished numerous field experiments and published their results along with his conclusions in three volumes entitled *A Course of Experimental Agriculture* (1771). Young insisted that experiments must be comparative. Further, he recognized the problem of bias in the investigator and warned investigators about inferring that results in a sample also apply to a wider population (Cochran, 1976).

At Rothamsted, Fisher studied voluminous past reports on the long sequence of yields of wheat from 13 parallel plots on Broadbalk field. Through his analyses of plot designs, he learned about randomization, replication, and other formerly unrecognized principles that could ensure both the efficiency of an experimental design and the validity of conclusions drawn from it. Fisher realized that conclusions reached by comparing the crop yields from two halves (plots A and B) of one field treated with different types of manure were invalid because field errors resulting from other variables (heterogeneous soil, texture, drainage, fertility, and microflora) that also affect crop yield were not considered.

> An estimate of the difference between plots A and B that could occur by chance alone in our experimental field, could have been obtained by comparing the yields of the halves during a number of previous seasons when they had been treated alike, but it would have taken an inordinately long time to reach an adequate estimate by this means. Ten years seemed minimal. [Box, 1978, p. 142]

As a more convenient device, Fisher adopted a common experimental practice and labeled it *replication* (He used more than the standard four or five replicates, however.)

> The experimental field was divided into a number of plots of equal size, and each treatment was assigned to several of the plots scattered over the whole area. The differences between plots treated differently then provided comparisons between treatments, while the differences between plots treated alike provided an estimate of their error. [Box, 1978, pp. 142–43]

Fisher later developed block plans that allowed for one replication of all treatments within each block. In this way, the blocks themselves could be in different fields or on different farms.

An experiment on potatoes culminated in a publication (Fisher and Mackenzie, 1923) in which Fisher began developing a three-way analysis of variance. "The experiment was actually of the split-plot type, for which Fisher's analysis was not fully correct. Evidently, he was feeling his way at that time" (Cochran, 1976). Fisher's analysis of variance table, however, saved much time and effort because it replaced lengthy calculations.

German economist Wilhelm Lexis had previously (1877) presented a mathematical theory for testing the homogeneity of a statistical series based on his work on the analysis of dispersion. Lexis's work anticipated Fisher's analysis of variance (Chang, 1976).

Between 1919 and 1925, in a series of articles broadly titled *Studies in Crop Variation* Fisher dealt with the analysis of variance and the principles of experimental design. "Within seven years he had solved all major problems and placed in the hands of the experimenter both the techniques for conducting experiments and the mathematical and arithmetical procedures for making sense of the results" (Box, 1978, p. 100).

As his work developed and his articles on crops, yields, rainfall, fertilizers, and the arrangements of field experiments were published, Fisher gradually came to be recognized as an expert researcher and statistician. He was consulted by many investigators in various areas— industry, medicine, forestry, horticulture, etc. Many voluntary workers came to Rothamsted to learn, and some stayed for months or years.

Statistical Methods for Research Workers (1925)

Fisher's first book, *Statistical Methods for Research Workers* (1925), has been published in English, French, German, Italian, Japanese, Spanish, and Russian and has undergone 13 updated editions as well as reprintings; it summarizes the principles of the statistical methods he developed at Rothamsted.

In the book, Fisher presented the statistical methods needed to design a proper trial, to analyze the results, and to draw appropriate conclusions that would have the assurance of validity. He deliberately did not emphasize theory, however, and did not generally present the mathematical derivations of formulas, leading later theoretical statisticians to say that they learned statistics by "reading between the lines" in Fisher.

As stated in the title of this chapter, the book (and Fisher at Rothamsted) represented the time and place when researchers and statisticians came together. (They had undoubtedly come together in Fisher's mind much earlier.) The debut of his book, however, was not auspicious.

His volume did not receive a single good review. The generous space given to Fisher's own work was criticized, as was the paucity of references to other statistical papers. His conclusions were considered to be still in the controversial stage (Box, 1978, p. 130). Soon after publication, however, he received a letter from a professor in Michigan "welcoming the book with a warmth of appreciation that touched Fisher like a ray of sunshine" (Box, 1978, p. 131).

This was not the first time that an original offering by Fisher had been scorned by some of his peers. Evidently, he developed his own practical philosophy about the acknowledgment to be expected from scientific achievements because he later said: "Recognition in science, to the man who has something to give, is, I should guess, more just and more certain than in most occupations but it does take time. And when it comes it will probably come from abroad" (Box, 1978, p. 131).

The Genetical Theory of Natural Selection (1930)

During the 1920s when Fisher was producing an astounding number of articles from Rothamsted data, he continued to write on genetics and eugenics. As a young man, he had readily accepted Charles Darwin's concept that, given variation, higher organisms had developed from lower ones through the process of natural selection of those best adapted to survive. His own studies on human inheritance led Galton to search for statistical methods that would enable him to analyze his observational data on continuous variables in humans. After reading Galton's *Natural Inheritance*, Weldon had concentrated on collecting measurements of body parts of many crustaceans and had taken his voluminous accumulation of figures to Karl Pearson for help with mathematical analysis. Fisher continued the chain of knowledge with his 1918 paper on the correlation between relatives, and this led to his further investigation of the dominance ratio found in the analyses of human measurements. In his 1922 article, *On the Dominance Ratio*, Fisher used a mathematical approach to explain a number of observed results:

1.   Gene frequencies are kept in stable equilibrium if the heterozygote (Aa) has a selective advantage over both homozygotes, either

AA (dominant) or aa (recessive). Thus, the mixed pair of genes (Aa) accumulates in the population while the others are eliminated. This explains why such genes are commonly found and may explain in part why inbreeding is sometimes detrimental.

2. The rate of mutation required to preserve the variability of a population is much lower than many biologists had assumed and, if selection were lacking, would be extremely small. Also, when a gene exists in a large number of individuals, even if they represent only a small proportion of the total population, chance will play little part in determining the gene's survival. Since natural selection expelled those genes that had striking or extreme effects, Fisher expected that "factors affecting important adaptations will be individually of very slight effect. We should thus expect that variation in organs of adaptive importance should be due to numerous factors which individually are difficult to detect" (Fisher, 1922b).

Thus, Fisher's work showed that Darwin had been correct in proposing that evolution depended on the selection of small continuous variations.

3. ". . . the assumption that leads to the level of dominance ratio actually observed in man is one of 'selection maintained in equilibrium by occasional mutation'" (Box, 1978, p. 179). "The rate of mutation required varies as the variance in the species, but it diminishes as the number of individuals is increased" (Fisher, 1922b).

Fisher continued to explore genetical theories. He and biologist E. B. Ford worked together to collect observational data to show that

> if the variation within a species were due to rare and random mutations, . . . and not to mutations induced by the environment, then . . . the variability of different species would be proportional to their relative abundance, and the greater variability of common species would be apparent in the local samples from a uniform environment. [Box, 1978, p. 181]

Fisher and Ford explored the variation of pigmentation on the wings of several species of night-flying moths and showed that "variability was strongly correlated with abundance . . . and that the rare mutations by which variability was maintained were not adaptive but random changes" (Fisher and Ford, 1926; Box, 1978, p. 181). Their observations also suggested that selection took place "to favor the [dark] protective coloration of the females at the expense of the paler males" (Fisher and Ford, 1928; Box, 1978, p. 182).

Fisher's ideas and statistical data were developed in stages over many years as he investigated dominance, mutations, and gene ratios. The culmination was *The Genetical Theory of Natural Selection* published in 1930.

The Design of Experiments (1935)

Fisher began *The Design of Experiments* (1935) by stating that criticisms of experimental conclusions usually follow along two lines of thought: (1) the reasoning, the inferences, or the interpretation of the results were illogical or (2) the experiment was poorly designed or badly executed. Fisher considered these criticisms to be "two different aspects of the same whole, and that whole comprises all the logical requirements of the complete process of adding to natural knowledge by experimentation" (Fisher, 1935, pp. 1–3).

He planned the book to show experimenters how appropriate consideration in advance can usually prevent such censure. The chapters are designed to clarify the principles that should prevail in all experimentation and include some of Fisher's most successful designs. In each chapter he proposed a commonplace problem and proceeded to design an experiment to test that question; his procedure, in general, was applicable to other similar situations.

His first example is the cup of tea experiment: one afternoon, soon after arriving at Rothamsted, Fisher poured a cup of tea and offered it to the woman standing beside him. She refused, remarking that she preferred milk to be in the cup before the tea was added. Fisher could not believe that there would be any difference in the taste, and, when the woman's fiancé suggested that an experiment be performed, Fisher was eager. An immediate trial was organized. The woman correctly identified more than enough of those cups into which tea had been poured first to prove her case (Box, 1978, pp. 134–35).

Using this example, Fisher stated the terms of the experiment minutely and distinctly; predicted all possible results, ascertaining, by sensible reasoning, what probability should be assigned to each possible result under the assumption that the woman was guessing; and determined the smallness of the probability he would require before he would be willing to admit the demonstration of a positive result. He also discussed tests of significance (based on calculating the probability that an observed or greater difference could occur by chance alone) under a null hypothesis (the assumption that there is no difference in experimental outcomes between the groups being tested), considerations of randomization when the experiment involves items (like cups of tea) that cannot be prepared exactly alike each time, and methods to increase the sensitiveness of the experiment.

In other chapters, Fisher discussed replication, randomized blocks, Latin squares, factorial designs, and confounding. He outlined ways of designing trials to get the most information from each circumstance.

"I think that I am pretty Tough"

Fisher's work with the Eugenics Education Society led in 1932 to an invitation to become a member of the Medical Research Council's Committee on Human Heredity. In 1933, he succeeded Karl Pearson as Galton Professor of Eugenics (or Human Genetics, as it is called today) at University College.

Introducing genetics into the research program, he promptly began to investigate human blood groups, and, in 1934, gained the sponsorship of the Rockefeller Foundation for a human serology unit in his department.

> In 1943, Fisher interpreted the bewildering results obtained with the new Rh blood groups in terms of three closely linked genes, each with alleles, and predicted the discovery of two new antibodies and an eighth allele—all of which were identified soon after. Fisher's enthusiasm for blood group polymorphisms continued to the end of his life and he did much to encourage studies of associations of blood groups and disease. [Box, 1983]

Three other events in 1943 had a deeply felt effect on him: his election to the Balfour Chair of Genetics at Cambridge; separation from his wife after a marriage of 26 years; and the death of his son George, who was on active service with the Royal Air Force. After George's death, Fisher wrote to a friend:

> I found myself pretty badly prepared for the shock. . . . One goes about rather automatically at first. With respect to anything I used to enjoy, I find that I still have my doubts. However, I think that I am pretty tough so surely I can take it. [Box, 1978, p. 397]

After George's death, Fisher was often seen wearing his son's raincoat of Air Force blue.

His Legacy

Fisher's list of publications is long. During his most productive years (1920–40), he published about 120 articles in addition to three books and a set of tables (Kendall, 1963). "Over a period of half a century Fisher turned out an average of one paper every two months" (Gridgeman, 1971).

After spending the summers of 1931 and 1936 teaching in the United States and the winter of 1937–38 in India, Fisher began to value international meetings as a way of keeping in touch with former colleagues and strengthening friendships—old and new. He was very distressed in 1941 when he had to cancel a planned visit to the United States because the British authorities, for unknown reasons, refused his application for an exit permit. After World War II, Fisher traveled to international meetings of statistical, genetical, and biometric societies; was elected the founding president of the Biometric Society in 1947; and served other statistical and genetical societies in their turn. He was knighted in 1952 and was president of the Royal Statistical Society in 1953–54.

Fisher spent the last years of his life in Australia, working in the Division of Mathematical Statistics of the Commonwealth Scientific and Industrial Research Organization (Gridgeman, 1971). He died in Adelaide on July 29, 1962, as the result of an embolism following surgery for cancer of the bowel; he had undergone the operation with only a local anesthetic (Reid, 1982, p. 257).

Many students today probably think of Fisher as the statistician who first proposed randomization as a procedure for unbiased assignment of treatments. In fact, Greenwood and Yule had discussed random allocation earlier in relation to trials of antityphoid and anticholera vaccines, but the method had not been used with subjects in any of the series they described. "The inoculated men volunteered, they were not selected at random" (Greenwood and Yule, 1915).

Fisher's contribution was the demonstration that randomization of treatments to the experimental units provides the physical basis for the validity of a test of statistical significance. That is, randomization of treatments makes it possible to calculate the probability that the observed or greater difference in outcomes between treatment groups is entirely related to chance, under the assumption of the null hypothesis that there is no real difference between the treatments.

Lachin (1988) wrote that "clinically and statistically, randomization is the single characteristic that most sharply distinguishes the controlled clinical trial from other forms of scientific investigation in medicine."

Randomization Involving Human Volunteers

While Fisher developed randomization to draw valid conclusions from field trials and other kinds of experiments, the format was soon put to use in the early clinical trials in England and the United States. In 1931, Amberson *et al.* of the Detroit Municipal Tuberculosis Sanatorium described a new drug treatment to selected patients and asked for volunteers; no mention was made of a control group. Twenty-four patients were chosen and, on the basis of clinical, laboratory, and x-ray findings, were divided into two approximately comparable groups of 12 each. The cases were individually matched. Then, by a flip of a coin, one group became identified as group I (recipients of sanocrysin, sodium-gold-thiosulfate) and the other as group II (control). Sanocrysin was given by injection; control patients received injections of distilled water. Participants were not told whether they were being treated with the active drug (Meinert, 1986, p. 6). Thus, possibly for the first time, the precept of single blindness was used in a clinical trial.

Seven years passed before the technique of randomization was used to assign individual patients to treatment. In a double-blind trial, Diehl *et al.* (1938) randomly allocated University of Minnesota volunteer students to one of three vaccines for the common cold or to placebo. All students thought that they were receiving a vaccine, and even physicians who saw the students at the health service when they contracted colds had no information about which group the student represented. A total of 1640 participants completed the trial.

These two publications are rarely mentioned in the literature; most statisticians remember Bradford Hill as the early proponent of randomization in medical trials. Since the early days of analyzing birth and death registrations, the British have been the acknowledged leaders in the fields of theoretical and practical statistics, and Bradford Hill continued that tradition. He designed the first clinical trial in which random numbers were used to assign participants to experimental and control groups, and over many years was in the forefront of medical statistics, particularly in the fields of clinical trials, public health, and ethics.

Sir Austin Bradford Hill (1897–1991)

"Random" Does Not Mean Haphazard

Bradford Hill (called Tony by his friends) might be described as a team player. He began his working career by cooperating with physicians and researchers, understanding that physicians are uneasy about withholding treatment or using placebos and agreeing that a physician has an overriding responsibility to a patient even if that means removing the patient from a comparative group. He was willing to accept that "while such removals may seriously weaken, or even destroy, the value of a trial, there [could] be no other means of meeting the ethical situation" (Hill, 1963).

On the other hand, he wrote, "In the assessment of a treatment medicine always has proceeded, and always must proceed, by way of experiment" (Hill, 1963). Hill quoted and agreed with an editor of the *British Medical Journal* who wrote, "In treating patients with unproved remedies we are, whether we like it or not, experimenting on human beings, and a good experiment well reported may be more ethical and entail less shirking of duty than a poor one" (Editor, *Br Med J* 2:1088–90, 1951; Hill, 1952). Hill also commended McCance (1951) who pointed out that "the medical profession has a responsibility not only for the cure of the sick and for the prevention of disease but for the advancement of knowledge upon which both depend. This third responsibility can be met only by investigation and experiment" (Hill, 1952).

Early on, in his relations with clinical physicians, Hill explained effectively and in a conciliatory manner that the word *random* did not mean haphazard, careless, or indiscriminate. Hill's modesty (he often wrote of himself as a layperson), his code of honor, and his willingness to accept a full share of the ethical responsibility in a clinical trial all contributed to his very successful professional life.

"Sir Austin's Career Did Not Begin Well"

Austin Bradford Hill was born in London in 1897, the third of six children. His father, Sir Leonard Erskine Hill, was a prominent physician, recognized for his work in physiology research (Hill, 1968).

In 1915, nearly 18 years old and due to be called up for military service at the age of 19, Bradford Hill decided to apply for a commission

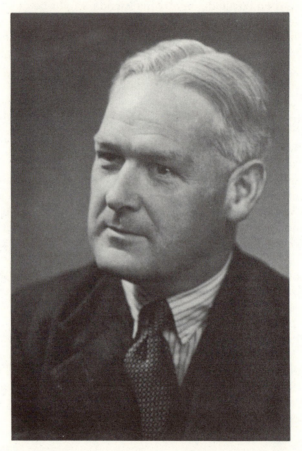

Sir Austin Bradford Hill. (From Dedication to Sir Austin Bradford Hill. 1982. *Stat Med* **1**(4), facing overleaf. Photograph taken by Bassano Studios/Elliott and Fry. Courtesy of the Royal Statistical Society.)

in His Majesty's service. At that time, Britain had no Air Force, but the Army had its own Royal Flying Corps and the Navy its Royal Naval Air Service. The Army was very "choosy" and, being deaf in one ear (from measles in childhood), Hill applied with the Navy. During the examination of his hearing, the medical officer whispered a number a fraction of a second before his assistant covered Hill's good ear, and the recruit satisfied requirements.

"In learning to fly the philosophy of the day was that a little wind was a dangerous thing" (Hill, 1983). With winter weather and the restriction of "no wind," it took 12 weeks to achieve only 6 hours of actual, spasmodic flying. Hill was dispatched on a solo circuit after 8 flying hours spread over 16 weeks.

A crash in 1916 was mentioned 65 years later when the Duke of Edinburgh conferred an honorary fellowship of the London School of Hygiene and Tropical Medicine:

> Sir Austin's career did not begin well. He made his first, rather negative, contribution to the public health as a Sublieutenant in the Royal Navy Air Service in the first world war. He somehow succeeded in polluting London's water supply by crash-landing one of His Majesty's aircraft into a major reservoir. He then served in the Aegean, where he gallantly but unsuccessfully attempted to drop a bomb on the enemy fleet. Unfortunately, the string attaching the bomb to his aircraft was knotted and the Navy was cheated of another famous victory. [Hill, 1983]

While in service Hill traveled to Paris, Rome, and the Greek islands, where he developed a chronic cough and malaise. Five months after his arrival in the Aegean in June 1917, Hill was diagnosed with tuberculosis and sent home to die. Because he was judged to have so little chance for survival, he was given a 100% disability pension for life. Hill survived a lung abscess, an artificial pneumothorax, and nearly 2 years of being bedbound (Hill, 1983).

> During long convalescence it was realized that his aim to take a medical qualification would not be practicable, so he studied for a London External degree in economics by correspondence course, chosen as the only subject even on the verge of science that could be done without any practical work. Having successfully taken this degree, he abandoned the study of economics and was offered a post with the Industrial Fatigue Research Board which was under the auspices of the Medical Research Council.
>   On the strength of this he married in 1923. His service with the

Board, investigating health problems in the cotton industry, among others, gave him his early training in epidemiology. In 1927 at the opening of the London School of Hygiene and Tropical Medicine, Major Greenwood was appointed as Professor of Epidemiology and Vital Statistics and took Hill onto his staff.

To learn some statistics, Hill attended lectures at University College London by Karl Pearson. When Greenwood retired in 1945, Hill was appointed to succeed him. [I. D. Hill, 1982]

Hill graduated from University College, London, with a B.S. degree in 1922, a Ph.D. degree in 1926, and a D.Sc. degree in 1929. From 1923 to 1932, he worked for the Industrial Health Research Board and Medical Research Council, and from 1932 to 1945 he was a reader in epidemiology and vital statistics at the London School of Hygiene and Tropical Medicine, where he was a professor of medical statistics from 1945 to 1961. During this latter period, Hill was also the honorary director of the Medical Research Council's Statistical Research Unit. He was president of the Royal Statistical Society from 1950 to 1952 and won their gold medal award in 1953.

Principles of Medical Statistics

In 1925, Hill published research on the average longevity of physicians. Using data in the roll of the Royal College of Physicians (London) from the beginning of the 17th century, he found that the expectation of life at ages 35 and over for all English males born between 1810 and 1875 was inferior to the expectation of physicians of the Royal College born over 100 years earlier. In a 1929 article, praised by Greenwood and Yule, Hill reported on illnesses occurring in various industrial occupations, and at a 1936 meeting of the Royal Statistical Society, he presented a comprehensive account of death rates from phthisis in England and Wales from 1851 to 1930 that showed a worrisome increase in the mortality rate for young adults.

About the same time, the editors of *Lancet* recognized that more and more of their articles contained statistical analyses of results, and that the methods and terms used were often perplexing to their readers, primarily physicians, who collected data haphazardly and did not understand statistical techniques or terms (Hill, 1937, foreword). Thus, in 1936, the *Lancet* editors invited Hill to prepare a series of articles concerning statistical methods. Hill wrote 17 articles that were published under the heading *Principles of Medical Statistics* from January through April 1937. The articles were short and concise and discussed the aim of the statistical method; selection; presentation of statistics; variability of observations; problems of sampling, including proportions, differences, and chi-square; the coefficient of correlation; life tables and survival after treatment; common fallacies and difficulties, including the crude death rate; general summary and conclusions; and calculations of standard deviation and the correlation coefficient. After the series was published, the *Lancet* editors wrote that Hill had exceeded their expectations. They believed that:

> whoever is writing an article, preparing a university thesis, planning a series of experiments, contemplating the issue of a questionnaire, or [worrying about] deductions from a sample typical (he hopes) of a larger population will gain from [studying them]; and most of all, perhaps, [such study will benefit] the doctor anxious to use the opportunities of general practice to solve some clinical or epidemiological problem. [Editors, *Lancet* 1:1473, 1937].

The articles were collected into a book (Hill, 1937), which, by 1993, had undergone 12 editions with appropriate face-lifts. The book continues to be well read by those desiring information on statistical methods, relating not only to medicine but to all sciences.

The Medical Research Council

When the United Kingdom Medical Research Council was organized, a department in the National Institute for Medical Research handled the statistical work. The group was later expanded by the addition of a small staff called the Statistical Committee. The department and the Statistical Committee were consolidated into the Statistical Research Unit in 1927 (Thomson, 1973). Hill coordinated and directed this staff from 1945 to 1961.

Because Hill worked primarily in public health, he often designed trials that involved communicable diseases, vaccines, and hazards in the workplace.

During the late 1930s, Hill worked on a research project in which ten generations of mice were inoculated with a partially purified toxic fraction isolated from *Bacillus typhimurium*, with each succeeding generation being bred from the survivors. This selective process produced a stock with a substantially increased power of resistance to the toxin and demonstrated the inheritance of resistance (Hill *et al.*, 1940).

In 1942, Britain began an immunization campaign against diphtheria. By 1947, it was apparent that poliomyelitis sometimes occurred soon after the injection of the diphtheria antigen. Hill and Knowelden (1950) analyzed 410 such cases of poliomyelitis. In 164 cases, records were obtained from closely paired children who had contracted poliomyelitis by other means (control group). The children inoculated within the month preceding the onset of poliomyelitis experienced paralysis in the limb that was the site of the diphtheria injection (usually the left arm) much more frequently than children in the control group. (In poliomyelitis, legs are usually affected two to three times as often as arms.)

Because many people in England believed that epidemics of poliomyelitis inordinately occurred in upper-class neighborhoods, Hill and Martin (1949) investigated poliomyelitis and the social environment. They showed that favorable social conditions in a locality need not raise fears of an unduly heavy risk of a polio epidemic.

In 1949, Hill's public health research also involved linking maternal rubella to congenital defects, but he and Galloway (1949) were unable to associate the two because of a lack of data from National Health Insurance files (Hill and Galloway). By 1958, however, Hill *et al.* were able to state that there was no evidence that mumps or measles (rubeola) during pregnancy had any deleterious effect on a fetus, that chicken pox might result in low birth weight, and that rubella that occurred early in a pregnancy could lead to congenital defects that involved the heart, vision, or hearing. The incidence of having an affected child was 50% if the mother contracted rubella during the first month of pregnancy, declining to 25% and 17% if the mother contracted rubella during the second and third months, respectively.

Gregg (1941) had reported that mothers of children with congenital cataract had frequently suffered from rubella during pregnancy, and many other physicians had substantiated the link between the effect of having that viral infection early in pregnancy and specific abnormalities in offspring (Doll, 1964). The data presented, however, were heavily biased because women who had children with birth defects readily reported whether they had had rubella during pregnancy but women with normal children rarely informed authorities about whether they had had rubella. Hill and colleagues' (1958) prospective cohort study, however, investigated the health of mothers during pregnancy and proceeded forward from notification of an attack of rubella to observe the proportion of the subsequent children born with defects.

Besides studying communicable diseases, Hill also researched health hazards in the workplace. In 1947, he cooperated in a study on the risk of contracting fluorosis to those who worked in magnesium factories. The investigation revealed an increased urinary excretion of fluorine in foundry workers compared with two control groups. Although only one worker had radiologic evidence of increased bone density, the researchers believed that at least some of the foundry workers were exposed to a risk of fluorosis and that production methods should be improved to reduce atmospheric contamination by fluorine compounds (Bowler *et al.*, 1947).

In 1948, Hill and Faning found a significant excess of deaths from cancer in factory workers handling inorganic compounds of arsenic.

Clinical Trials

The need for clinical trials became obvious to the Medical Research Council in the early 1930s, and in 1931, an announcement in *Lancet* noted that a therapeutic trials committee had been organized to advise and assist in arranging properly controlled clinical testing of new products that showed potential for treating disease (Medical Research Council, 1931; Meinert, 1986, p. 7). The format of using many investigators from different locations who conformed to the same study protocol for a clinical trial appeared around the late 1930s and early 1940s. One of the early examples of this arrangement was a study of the common cold (Patulin Clinical Trials Committee, 1944; Meinert, 1986, p. 7).

> None of the early evaluations of penicillin involved controls. The dramatic recoveries achieved in treating infections, theretofore fatal, were by themselves sufficient to establish the efficacy of the treatment. [Meinert, 1986, p. 5; Keefer *et al.*, 1943]

Hill (1950) confirmed the importance of a placebo treatment in a clinical trial on the efficacy of antihistamines against the common cold. Daily records were available for 1156 volunteers having colds; 579 patients were taking antihistamines and 577 were taking a placebo. After the second day of treatment, the proportions of cured and improved patients in the antihistamine group were 8.8 and 53.0%, respectively. Unfortunately, this seemingly positive result on the efficacy of antihistamines was contradicted by similar results (8.5% of patients cured and 51.3% of patients showing improvement) from the placebo group. The study was important, however, because it was one of the earliest studies to use the double-blind technique, which means that neither the patient nor the researcher knew whether the patient was being treated with an antihistamine or a placebo.

Doll and Hill's (1950) retrospective method of inquiry in their pioneer study establishing smoking as an important factor in the development of carcinoma of the lung became a prototype for later case–control designs. Their 1950 publication was followed by others (Hill and Doll, 1956, 1960; Hill, 1957) as the two continued to present facts and statistics on the relationship between tobacco and lung cancer.

In a preventive medicine study (Medical Research Council, 1951), Hill devised a plan of assignment by random order for 6710 British children who participated in a clinical trial from 1946 to 1950 in which they were inoculated with either *Haemophilus pertussis* vaccine or anti-catarrhal vaccine. After some follow-up time, whooping cough was diagnosed in 149 children vaccinated with *H. pertussis* and in 687 children vaccinated with anticatarrhal. The trial showed that inoculation with the *H. pertussis* vaccine reduced the incidence of whooping cough by 78%.

In 1946, Hill also had the opportunity to use random sampling numbers to assign treatment in the first strictly controlled clinical trial. In that year, the Medical Research Council began planning a study of the efficacy of streptomycin against progressing bilateral pulmonary tuberculosis. Streptomycin had been discovered in 1944, and in a few clinical experiments, physicians had reported positive results. The drug was marketed in the United States, but little money was available in postwar England, and researchers were limited to a small amount. This created an excellent opportunity for Hill, who had been anxious to plan a randomized clinical study with controls (Hill, 1990). Under ordinary circumstances, it would have been unethical to withhold available treatment from very ill patients, but the Medical Research Council considered that it would be unethical not to seize the opportunity to design a strictly controlled clinical trial that could evaluate the efficacy of streptomycin therapy expediently (Hill, 1963).

For each recruiting hospital in the study, Hill drew up random sampling numbers for each sex. These were contained in a set of sealed envelopes identified only by the hospital name and a number on the outside. After a patient was accepted for the study, the appropriate numbered envelope was opened at the central office, and the physician was told whether that subject would receive streptomycin plus bed rest (55 patients, streptomycin group) or the current therapy of bed rest only

(52 patients, control group). All of the participating patients were admitted to hospitals during 1947. Streptomycin therapy was stopped after 4 months. After 6 months, 4 (7%) of the streptomycin patients and 14 (27%) of the control patients had died; after 1 year, 12 (22%) of the streptomycin patients and 24 (46%) of the control patients had died. This latter difference in mortality rates is statistically significant. G. B. Hill (1983) pointed out that the "statistical analyses, though cogent and detailed, are simple and descriptive. Formal statistical testing is used only twice—to test the difference between the response and fatality rates in the treated and [in] the controls."

In this streptomycin experiment, patients were not told that they were entering a clinical trial or that they would get special treatment. No consent forms were used, and throughout the hospital stay, control patients were not told that they were controls in a study (Medical Research Council, 1948). "The details of the series were unknown to any of the investigators or to the coordinator" (Marshall and Merrell, 1949).

The study became a prototype for therapeutic testing, and Hill's criteria for designing trials gained wide recognition. He later stated (1963) that

> whenever a newly introduced drug or vaccine is scarce in its early days, then there presents an opportunity of which immediate advantage should, if possible, be taken. With a serious disease in which the old offers very little hope of benefit the new cannot be withheld. The chance of adequately and quickly assessing the value of the latter, if any, may never again occur.

In Hill's inaugural address as president of the Royal Statistical Society, he reviewed the Health Service Act of 1948 and the National Health Insurance Act. Under the fitting title *The Doctor's Day and Pay* (Hill, 1951a), he discussed the consequences of a physician's income depending on his A's (attendance of patients at the physician's surgery) and V's (visits by the physician to the insured patients).

After the streptomycin study, he participated in numerous randomized clinical studies, collaborating with physicians on trial design and analysis.

An Uncommon Degree of Common Sense

Throughout his career Hill wrote extensively about clinical trial design, analysis techniques, and ethical considerations. Popular papers included *The Clinical Trial* (1951b, 1952), *Observation and Experiment* (1953), and *Medical Ethics and Controlled Trials* (1963). In *The Environment and Disease: Association or Causation?* (1965) he reminded readers that tests of significance were being overdone in the medical literature. He stated that there were innumerable situations where such tests were totally unnecessary and that "we weaken our capacity to interpret data and to take reasonable decisions whatever the value of P."

The use of confidence intervals has become more widespread since Hill's article was written. He often spoke out, however, for readers to give more consideration to thoughtful evaluation of publication results. He urged them to assess the hypothesis being tested, search for evidence of partiality or bias, and use clinical judgment in accepting or rejecting the findings. He wrote, "Like fire, the chi-square test is an excellent servant and a bad master" (Hill, 1965).

In *Reflections on the Controlled Trial* (1966) Hill stressed that each trial must be designed so that researchers will be in a position to generalize from the results—in other words, that the treatment is of value for a certain type of patient, and not just for the particular participating group. He also explained how the double-blind study frequently hampers the clinician in making discriminating observations concerning his patient.

Speaking to the British Committee on the Safety of Drugs, Hill commented that no committee of this kind can wait until every "i" has been dotted and every "t" crossed:

> It has to walk a wobbly rope, balancing between panicking over something that is suggestive but may turn out to be unimportant and doing nothing because the case is unproven and yet may turn out to be true so that harm is meanwhile done. [Hill, 1971]

Sir Austin Hill often wrote letters to medical journals, using a published article to make a point about clinical trial technique. In one such communication he recommended using a variable-dose design and then outlined the design's salient features (Hill, 1982). In another, he wrote that randomization does not contribute to the ethical problem inherent in a trial but is merely a technique for producing two groups in an unbiased way and securing, as far as possible, their comparability. The ethical problem is whether or not the investigator is entitled to use patients in the protocol he has proposed. He must first face that problem and make his decision; randomization comes in later (Hill, 1987).

Often, Hill wrote these letters quite late in his life; he had a very active mind, even well into his eighties. It appears that he stayed involved and maintained his spirit and interest to a ripe old age.

Sir Harold Himsworth (1982) wrote that physicians with no flair for mathematics were relieved to hear Hill state that he himself always relied on simple arithmetic. Of course, this was an exaggeration, but Hill was not schooled in theoretical mathematics.

In 1959, while spending a year at the London School of Hygiene and Tropical Medicine, the first lecture that Marvin Schneiderman of the National Cancer Institute attended was a talk by Hill on controlled experiments. Hill concluded by asking, "See that American back there in the back row? Did you know that he is the father of twins? Had one baptized and saved the other for a control" (Schneiderman, 1982).

Sir Austin Bradford Hill died April 18, 1991; his wife had died in 1980. He is survived by two sons and a daughter.

CHAPTER 4

The Awakening of Statistics
in the United States

The American Statistical Association (ASA)

On November 27, 1839, five men—Rev. William Cogswell, John Dix
Fisher, M.D., the Honorable Richard Fletcher, Oliver W. B. Peabody, and
Lemuel Shattuck—met in Boston to found a statistical organization;
they called it the American Statistical Society. During the following year,
a constitution and a new name, the American Statistical Association
(with a preferable abbreviation), were approved (Mason *et al.*, 1990). The
group's expressed purpose was to accumulate and classify data from
many areas of concern; little attention was given to the mathematics
required for meaningful analysis. An early letter to members shows
that the ASA was interested in receiving reports on topography, population, education, associations, the press, government, public defense,
casualties, crime, pauperism, benevolence, and religion (Historical exhibits, 1940; M. Anderson, 1989).

The membership of the ASA in the early years (never more than 75
people) was centered in Boston; usually, 10 or fewer members attended
quarterly meetings. "Statists," as they were called then, were self-
taught, although colleges began to supply elementary training in interpreting data around 1880. The ASA meetings provided a time and place
to come together for discussions, during which rules were created and
adopted for data collection, classification, presentation, and analysis.
Scientific papers were presented at each meeting, and all full members

were required to have at least one paper ready to deliver; most reports included demographic or social data (Mason *et al.*, 1990). Members also served as lobbyists, and one statist lobbied successfully for the first individual-level census in the United States, which was accomplished in Boston in 1845 (M. Anderson, 1989). Between 1865 and 1889, they lobbied for adoption of the metric system in the United States (Mason *et al.*, 1990).

Some ASA members met with governmental officials in charge of statistics and offered advice on improving data gathering, classification, and publication. Edward Jarvis, M.D., the third president of the ASA, recognized the misrepresentation of blacks and the insane in the 1840 U.S. census; he became a consultant on the censuses of 1850, 1860, and 1870. Despite these links of communication with the national government, the ASA was really limited in locale because most of the members lived in the New England states, predominantly in the Boston area (Mason *et al.*, 1990). Jarvis was president for 31 years, but when Francis A. Walker succeeded him, things began to change.

General Francis Amasa Walker (1840–1897)

Francis Walker, economist and president of the Massachusetts Institute of Technology (MIT), served as president of the ASA from 1883 to 1896 and vowed to expand the influence of the statistical association; he believed that it should be a national society. His recording secretary, Davis R. Dewey, was charged with initiating the publication of a journal, and, in 1888, the first issue of *Publications of the American Statistical Association* appeared. The name was later changed to the *Journal of the ASA* (M. Anderson, 1989).

Walker was the foremost statistician of his day. He was appointed to oversee and direct the 1870 and 1880 federal censuses, and during his tenure, the ASA was influential in the creation of the Bureau of Labor Statistics (1885). On December 31, 1896, Walker journeyed to Washington, D.C., to speak at the first meeting of the ASA to be held in that city. Six days later, he died suddenly (Noether, 1989). By this time, the ASA had grown to 533 members (Mason *et al.*, 1990). Today, it serves more than 15,000 members.

In his last speech to the ASA, Walker criticized the United States for spending tens of millions of dollars on the collection and publication of statistical information without contributing any money to train and prepare the people who would conduct the statistical services of the country.

> . . . Our statistical work, national, state, and municipal, has fallen into hands, almost without exception, . . . of men with intelligence, with perhaps a very deep interest in their subject . . . but men who have had not only no training in statistical methods and statistical administration, but have also lacked that elementary knowledge of the subject which was necessary to save them from making great errors of judgment, and sometimes monstrous errors in their conclusions. . . . All those who have had anything to do with American statistics came into the service comparatively late in life, without any elementary training, sometimes taking up the most gigantic piece of work . . . simply with an interest in the subject as the only guarantee of their competence for the service. [F. A. Walker, 1897; Noether, 1989]

The Early Years of Teaching

The first documented use of the word *statistics* in a U.S. college catalog may have occurred when the University of Virginia listed a course in political economy, statistics, and the philosophy of social relations for its 1845–46 school year. The class was taught by the Rev. William Holmes McGuffey, famous for the widely used *McGuffey Readers* (Fitzpatrick, 1955; Noether, 1989).

Nearly 30 years later, in 1873–74, Francis Walker taught public finance and the statistics of industry at Yale University. During the 1880s, instruction in statistics was introduced at Columbia College, the Wharton School in Philadelphia, MIT, Johns Hopkins University, and the University of Michigan (Noether, 1989).

The content of the courses was typical of classes given on the European continent (Germany, France, and Italy), with emphasis on political arithmetic. During this period, several prominent men, Carroll D. Wright (commissioner of the Federal Bureau of Labor), Davis Dewey (assistant professor of economics and statistics at MIT), and Francis Walker, took every opportunity to exert pressure on academic leaders to include statistics in their college curricula (Wright, 1888; Dewey, 1889; F. A. Walker, 1890; Noether, 1989).

In 1902, a permanent Office of the Census was established, and, concurrently, more and more colleges and universities were initiating courses in statistics. Also Quetelet (from Belgium) and the British school of statisticians (Galton, Edgeworth, Karl Pearson, and their students) were gaining more authority and influence, and the textbooks of the first two decades of the 20th century reflected an emphasis on mathematics.

> There are now lengthy discussions of measures of central tendency and dispersion, of symmetry and skewness, of correlation and association, of smoothing time series and constructing index numbers. For each new quantity, there are detailed instructions on how to carry out the required calculations. And in a few advanced texts we begin to find references to probable errors and hypothesis testing. [Noether, 1989]

In 1926, Glover reported results of a questionnaire on statistics instruction. At the 125 institutions that responded, elementary statistics was offered by about 60% of economics departments, 40% of the schools of business, and 30% of the departments of public health, psychology, and agriculture. About 30% of the mathematics departments taught advanced statistics. At many schools, the center of statistics instruction had moved from departments of economics to mathematics, and subsequently, this resulted in a concentration on mathematical, rather than statistical, ideas. Statistics came to be regarded as simply a branch of mathematics (Noether, 1989).

Henry Lewis Rietz (1875–1943)

Henry Rietz received his Ph.D. degree from Cornell University in 1902. He settled at the University of Iowa at Iowa City in 1918 and was very active during the period when ideas conceived in Europe were being introduced in the United States.

His monograph, *Mathematical Statistics*, appeared in 1927 and had its fifth printing in 1947. Probably some people who read the book went to the University of Iowa to become Rietz's students, and a number of his students went on to become well-known scholars. A few of these prominent men were Allen T. Craig, Rietz's successor at Iowa; Carl F. Fischer at the University of Michigan; and Samuel S. Wilks at Princeton.

In 1935, the Institute of Mathematical Statistics (IMS) was formed with Rietz as president. Annual dues were five dollars and included a subscription to the IMS's official journal, the *Annals of Mathematical Statistics*, created by Harry C. Carver in 1930 (Neyman, 1976).

Harry C. Carver (1890–1977)

Around 1910, Professor J. W. Glover, who had started the actuarial program at the University of Michigan, decided that courses in mathematical statistics should be included. In 1916, he recruited Harry Carver, a recent graduate, to develop such courses. As late as 1922, there were only two schools in the United States (Iowa State College and the University of Michigan) that offered classes in mathematical statistics (Craig, 1986).

Carver was a young instructor, and his first classes (Mathematics 49 and 50), each for 2-hour credits, were at a precalculus level (Craig, 1986). He used Yule's *An Introduction to the Theory of Statistics* supplemented with writings from Karl Pearson, Student, Fisher, and others (Neyman, 1976).

Carver's classes generated papers concerned with mathematical statistics, but he eventually complained to the ASA about the problem of finding editors who would accept these manuscripts. The officials of the ASA were understanding but explained that their membership included primarily bankers, economists, and census workers who knew little mathematics. Also, mathematical formulas would require expensive monotype composition, rather than the cheaper linotype then in use (Neyman, 1976). Therefore, like Karl Pearson and Weldon before him, Carver started his own journal—the *Annals of Mathematical Statistics*, which first appeared in February 1930. Carver assumed financial responsibility for the new journal and served as its editor until 1935, when *Annals* became the official publication for the newly created IMS. At that time, *Annals* apparently filled a need because it had subscriptions from 118 individuals and 98 libraries (Neyman, 1976).

An adequate supply of articles was submitted to *Annals* for publication, but the scarcity of funds to meet publication needs was worrisome. At times toward the end of World War II, the journal almost went bankrupt. C. C. Craig later wrote (1986), "I don't know if Carver ever told anybody the cost in dollars of his devotion to statistics but I doubt if he knew closely." Fortunately, the officials at the journal and at the IMS had accumulated a large inventory of back issues during the war, and once the war was over, there was a sizable demand for them. Paul Dwyer and Carl Fischer handled these transactions, and their hard work brought in enough money to establish a sound financial base for the *Annals* (Craig, 1986). The journal grew and in 1973 was replaced by two periodicals: the *Annals of Statistics* and the *Annals of Probability* (Neyman, 1976). In 1986, *Statistical Science* was founded; its role, as stated in the journal, is to present the full range of contemporary statistical thought at a technical level accessible to a broad community of practitioners, teachers, researchers, and students of statistics and probability.

George W. Snedecor (1881–1974)

After receiving an M.A. degree in physics from the University of Michigan in 1913, George Snedecor was hired to be an assistant professor of mathematics at Iowa State College of Agriculture and Mechanics, in Ames. He was promoted to associate professor in 1914 and, 1 year later, began teaching the first formal course in statistics (Bancroft, 1972) called Mathematics as Applied to Social and Economic Problems (Lush, 1972).

Agriculture was the main industry in Iowa, and farming and animal husbandry became the focus of many college courses. Even today, Iowa's manufacturing output is directly related to its agricultural predominance; its main industries are food processing and manufacturing agricultural machinery. In 1924, Snedecor attended a 10-week seminar conducted by Henry A. Wallace (who later became vice president of the United States) on rapid machine calculation of correlation coefficients, partial correlation, and the calculation of regression lines. The following year, the two men coauthored a bulletin, *Correlation and Machine Calculations* (Wallace and Snedecor, 1925), which was distributed worldwide (Bancroft, 1972).

Wallace, an alumnus of Iowa State, was an editor with *Wallace's Farmer*, a newspaper founded by his grandfather. He asked Snedecor to organize Saturday afternoon meetings for research workers in agriculture (Bancroft, 1972). Wallace's father, Henry C. Wallace, was the Secretary of Agriculture from 1921 until his death in 1924, and Henry A. visited Washington frequently and became interested in the punch-card machines that were being used in the Federal Bureau of Agricultural Economics. He realized their laborsaving potential for statisticians: "Those who began their statistical apprenticeship later than the early 1920s can scarcely imagine the many hours previously spent by high-powered research men in the drudgery of computing correlation coeffi-

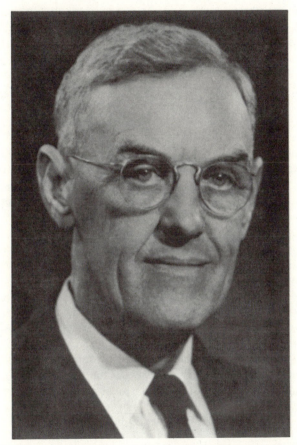

George W. Snedecor. (Reprinted by permission from *Statistical Papers in Honor of George W. Snedecor* by T. A. Bancroft. © Copyright 1972, by Iowa State University Press, Ames.)

cients one by one" (Lush, 1972). Wallace borrowed some card-handling equipment from an insurance company in Des Moines, hauling the machines back and forth each Saturday for the afternoon seminars.

Snedecor had acquired a card punch and verifier by 1924 when A. E. Brandt joined the college staff. The two of them started helping colleagues analyze research data. They would take the punched cards to Des Moines and use a sorter and tabulator at the insurance company. The success and inconvenience of this led to the creation of the Mathematics Statistical Service in 1927 with Snedecor and Brandt in charge. As part of this service, the college installed IBM card sorting and tabulating machines for the first time (Lush, 1972).

In 1931, Snedecor became a professor of mathematics, and the first degree in statistics at Iowa State (a Master's of Science) was awarded to his student, Gertrude M. Cox (Bancroft, 1972).

Because Snedecor recognized the importance of Sir Ronald Fisher's work, Iowa State was the first U.S. college to acknowledge the accomplishments of the British statistician and to grant him an honorary degree. Fisher was a visiting lecturer on the Iowa State campus during the summers of 1931 and 1936 (Bancroft, 1972).

From 1933 to 1947, Snedecor was the director of the Statistical Laboratory at Iowa State. The Department of Statistics was created in 1947, but Snedecor was never its official head (Lush, 1972). From 1947 to 1958, he was a professor of statistics.

In 1948, Snedecor became president of the ASA; he was the first president to be selected from the field of agricultural research. His best-known publication, *Statistical Methods*, appeared in 1937, with many subsequent editions.

Snedecor was instrumental in securing Iowa State's international reputation for leadership in statistics. In the early years, he "almost singlehandedly kept the United States abreast of developments in applied statistics" (Mood, 1990).

Gertrude M. Cox (1900–1978)

Born in Dayton, Iowa, at the beginning of the 20th century, Gertrude Cox followed the basic ethics of that time and place. In her day, children were expected to have high principles and good character; they learned that integrity, honesty, and trustworthiness were important attributes. Most of all, children were taught the value of hard work.

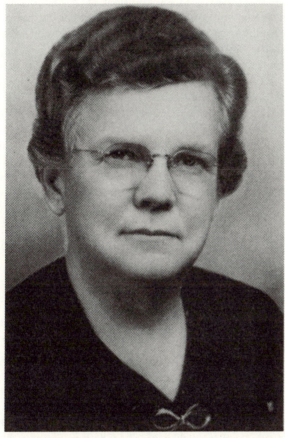

Gertrude M. Cox. (From Stinnett, S., and Collaborators, 1990, Women in statistics: Sesquicentennial activities. *Am Stat* **44**:75. Courtesy of the American Statistical Association.)

As is often the case with those who accomplish much in a lifetime, Cox seemed to set goals for herself at each stage of her career; she then worked tirelessly with unusual tenacity and independence to achieve each target. She would probably attribute her success to luck or to being in the right place at the right time, but the facts reveal that she prepared herself well so that she could fulfill each opportunity that came along.

As a young woman, she believed that her life's work should be as a deaconess in the Methodist Episcopal church, and she prepared for it, including spending some time caring for children in an orphanage in Montana (R. L. Anderson *et al.*, 1979). Cox changed her mind, however, and entered Iowa State College, earning a B.S. degree at the age of 29. As mentioned before, the first degree in statistics at Iowa State, an M.S., was awarded to Cox in 1931.

After she spent 2 years at the University of California at Berkeley, Snedecor hired Cox as a member of the small group that would be responsible for the newly created Statistical Laboratory at Iowa State. She worked there from 1933 to 1940. Cox always enjoyed telling about Snedecor's dedication of his book, *Statistical Methods*. "The dedication simply read, 'to Gertrude,' but Professor Snedecor never did specify to which Gertrude he referred—his wife Gertrude or his professional colleague Gertrude" (R. L. Anderson *et al.*, 1979).

William Cochran worked with Cox from 1938 to 1940 and wrote that, at that time, in addition to determining the appropriate statistical analyses for research projects, she was assembling material on experimental designs (Cochran, 1979). A book by that name was completed by Cochran and Cox and published in 1950.

> Since Gertrude disliked the job of writing even more than I did, she took responsibility for the experimental plans, and I took primary responsibility for the descriptive text and any hidden theory. Misprints and errors in the Cochran text have kept me busy at times for quite a number of years. In over 25 years, one misprint in one treatment in one plan has been brought to my attention. This performance was typical of Gertrude's work. The letter pointing out this misprint cheered me up no end. [Cochran, 1979]

Around 1940, North Carolina State College was preparing to inaugurate its new Department of Experimental Statistics in the School of Agriculture. Snedecor was asked to suggest names of qualified candidates for the unfilled position of head of the department. He showed his proposed list of men to Cox, who immediately asked, "Why didn't you put my name on the list?" A footnote was then added, "Of course, if you would consider a woman for this position, I would recommend Gertrude Cox of my staff" (R. L. Anderson et al., 1979). She was selected and spent the rest of her life in North Carolina.

She assumed additional responsibilities as the director of a new Institute of Statistics at North Carolina State in 1944. Cox secured new faculty members for North Carolina State (including Cochran), she recruited Harold Hotelling to head the new Department of Statistics at the University of North Carolina, and she assisted in organizing the Department of Biostatistics in the School of Public Health at Chapel Hill with Bernard G. Greenberg as its head (Stinnett, 1990).

Although each of her two executive positions at the college would have been a full-time task for any ordinary mortal, Cox continued to teach her intermediate experimental design course. Like Fisher's format in the *Design of Experiments*, she used real-life examples that she had accumulated from her years of consulting experience. Students from many academic fields took her class, and it was required for those majoring in statistics (R. L. Anderson et al., 1979). To her credit, she stimulated and encouraged many young scholars to pursue a career in statistics. She believed (again like Fisher) that statistics needed to be made practical for those working in agricultural and biologic research; she bridged the gap between theoreticians and research workers (Stinnett, 1990).

In the late 1950s, she was involved in planning the future Research Triangle Institute (RTI), which would integrate Duke University at Durham, the University of North Carolina at Chapel Hill, and North Carolina State at Raleigh.

She resigned from her two offices at North Carolina State College in 1960 to undertake the task of organizing and then becoming head of the Statistics Research Division at the RTI. After 5 years, she withdrew to a position as consultant to the RTI and to governmental agencies (Stinnett, 1990).

At this stage of her life, Cox embarked on extensive overseas travel (23 trips), concentrating especially on promoting statistical activities in Egypt and Thailand. On five separate occasions, she made lengthy visits to Thailand to work on their statistics programs. The Thais appreciated her interest and respected her abilities, always welcoming her back to her "second home" (R. L. Anderson et al., 1979). Cox also entertained a steady succession of visitors to her home in Raleigh.

She helped found the Biometric Society (1947) and the journal

Biometrics (first called *Biometrics Bulletin*), which she edited for 11 years. She served as president of the ASA in 1956 and of the Biometric Society for the 1968–69 year. In 1949, she became the first woman to be elected to the International Statistical Institute (ISI) (Stinnett, 1990).

She received many well-deserved honors and awards, including a doctor of science degree from Iowa State College in 1958; at North Carolina State University, Cox Hall was dedicated in 1970, and the Cox Fellowship Fund was established in 1977 (Stinnett, 1990).

Gertrude Cox died of leukemia in October 1978. A month later, a memorial service was held in Bangkok for this remarkable woman whom the Thais loved and admired (R. L. Anderson *et al.*, 1979).

Harold Hotelling (1895–1973)

Harold Hotelling was born in Fulda, Minnesota. He earned a B.A. degree in journalism and an M.A. degree in mathematics from the University of Washington and a Ph.D. degree in mathematics from Princeton University (1924). From 1924 to 1927, Hotelling worked in the Food Research Institute at Stanford University, where he assessed crop yields and essential nutrient conditions. In 1927, he was named associate professor of mathematics at Stanford and held that position until 1931. He took a 6-month leave of absence in 1929 to go to Rothamsted and study with Ronald A. Fisher (Hoeffding, 1978). This contact with Fisher proved to be an important influence on Hotelling's beliefs, career, and teaching methods. In addition, the sojourn in England helped to solidify his interest in mathematical statistics.

In 1931, he was selected to fill the position of professor of economics at Columbia University. He organized a set of courses in mathematical statistics, but there was no departmental structure, and he did not have degree-granting authority or scholarships (Arrow, 1988).

Hotelling remained at Columbia for 15 years, accomplishing his most important work during this period. His publications demonstrate a continuing interest in multivariate analysis as applied to mathematical economics and various fields of statistics. In his first significant paper about statistics, *The Generalization of Student's Ratio* (1931a), he derived what is now known as Hotelling's generalized T^2 test, which extends Student's test for the mean of a univariate normal distribution to multivariate situations (Hoeffding, 1978). The article was soon recognized as a valuable addition to statistical theory.

Hotelling was considered to be a pioneer in the areas of multivariate

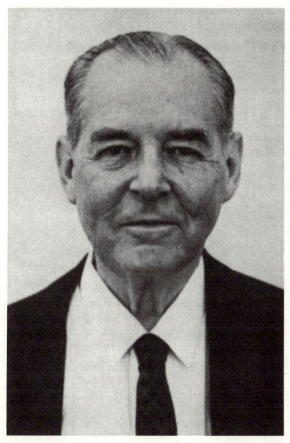

Harold Hotelling. (From Golden Oldies: Classic articles from the world of statistics and probability. 1988. *Stat Sci* **3**:64. Courtesy of the Institute of Mathematical Statistics.)

analysis, frequency distributions (1931b), component analysis (1933), canonical analysis (1936), and statistical prediction (1935, 1942a). He wrote the section on frequency distributions in the *Encyclopedia of the Social Sciences*, vol. 6 (1931b), and the foreword to *Tables of Probability Functions*, vol. II, for the National Bureau of Standards (1942b). His studies of differential equations subject to error (1927) and of the experimental determination of the maximum of a function (1941) stimulated considerable further research (W. L. Smith, 1978).

Like Fisher and Gertrude Cox, Hotelling often worked on practical problems that he encountered in his professional or personal life. For instance, another paper on multivariate analysis resulted from the issue of quality control in testing bombsights during World War II (Hotelling, 1947; Levene, 1974). Other examples include an unpublished research project (undertaken while he was a young journalism student employed by a local weekly) on the effect newspaper articles had on elections (Levene, 1974) and papers on birth rate variability (Hotelling and Hotelling, 1931) and the duration of pregnancy (Hotelling and Hotelling, 1932). The latter two, initiated by his first wife's pregnancies, were coauthored with her. She died in 1932.

Hotelling also became absorbed in improving efficiency in the use of desk calculators and punch card accounting machines. Levene, one of Hotelling's students, remembers:

> Even the evaluation of the normal integral did not escape his notice, and a lecture was devoted to obtaining it, so that "if you are ever stranded on a desert island without tables, you will be able to calculate normal curve probabilities." [Levene, 1974]

During World War II, Hotelling organized the Statistical Research Group, which applied its expertise to some projects directed by the National Defense Research Committee. While working as a consultant to this group, Abraham Wald developed his basic theory of sequential analysis and worked out the sequential probability ratio test (Wald, 1947) (see Chapter 6).

Hotelling was a spirited teacher. He concerned himself with the problems of young people and was always on the alert for exceptional talent, often finding it among Jewish scholars in New York or learned war refugees. "At a time when good positions in universities and industry went to WASPs [white Anglo-Saxon Protestants), he always supported the best qualified for each position" (Levene, 1974).

During the 1930s, Hotelling became very troubled about the competence of people who were teaching statistics, and "he was openly dissatisfied with the low status of statistics at Columbia or any other university" (Arrow, 1988). In many colleges, courses in statistics were offered in multiple departments (e.g., agriculture, anthropology, astronomy, biology, business, economics, education, engineering, psychology), and Hotelling found that, in many situations, the instructors were the departments' graduate students who had minimal knowledge of statistics (Neyman, 1976).

In 1940, Hotelling, as chairman of the Committee on the Teaching of Statistics of the IMS, had written the first of two articles as a position statement for the committee and presented it at an IMS meeting in September 1940. This was his classic paper, *The Teaching of Statistics*, and following his presentation there was a unanimous vote to publish it in the *Annals* as an expression of IMS opinion on the matter (Bradley, 1988). Hotelling wrote:

> The obvious inefficiency of overlapping and duplicating courses given independently in numerous departments by persons who are not really specialists in the subject leads to the suggestion that the whole matter be taken over by the Department of Mathematics. This is a promising solution, but it is doomed to failure if, as has sometimes happened, it means that the teaching of statistics is put under the jurisdiction of those who have no real interest in it. Moreover the teaching of statistics cannot be done appreciably better by mathematicians ignorant of the subject than by psychologists or agricultural experimenters ignorant of the subject. . . .
>
> The most essential thing [for a good teacher of statistics] is that the man shall know the theory of statistics itself thoroughly from the ground up, including the mathematical derivations of proper methods and a clear knowledge of how to apply them in various empirical fields. In addition, . . . a competent statistician or teacher of statistics needs a really intimate acquaintance with the problems of one or more empirical subjects in which statistical methods are applied. This is quite important. Sometimes excellent mathematicians have wasted time and misled students through failure to get that feeling for applications that is necessary for proper statistical work. . . .
>
> For efficient functioning of the institution as a whole it should be agreed that the Department of Statistics or the Department of Mathematics should do *all* the elementary instruction in statistics,

and that courses in statistics in other departments should be confined to applications of the basic theory.

Jerzy Neyman was so impressed by the speech that when he invited Hotelling to the 1945 Berkeley Symposium on Mathematical Statistics and Probability, he suggested that in addition to presenting a theoretical paper, Hotelling should also deliver a paper on *The Place of Statistics in the University* (Reid, 1982, p. 198). Hotelling addressed his concerns.

> Organization of the teaching of statistical methods should be centralized, and should provide also for the joint functions of research and of advice and service needed by others in the institution, and possibly outside it, regarding the statistical aspects of their problems of designing experiments and interpreting observations. Beginning courses in statistical methods and theory should be taught only under the supervision of the central statistical organization. . . . A vast amount of research, mostly of a highly mathematical character, is needed and is in prospect. Anyone who does not keep in active touch with this research will after a short time not be a suitable teacher of statistics. Unfortunately, too many people like to do their statistical work just as they say their prayers—merely substitute in a formula found in a highly respected book written a long time ago. [Hotelling, 1949]

Neyman believed that it was unwise to separate statistics from mathematics. "Such separation can produce practitioners of statistics who can apply such theory as they have learned and do useful substantive work, but they would probably not contribute to theory unless they filled in the gaps in their mathematical education" (Neyman, 1976). Nevertheless, Hotelling's ideas made an impression on the academic community and contributed to the creation of some of the first departments of statistics in U.S. universities (Hoeffding, 1978). Some prominent statisticians, however, believe that Hotelling's essays could have been written today because the same educational organization he argued against still exists in many institutions, and statistics has failed to achieve its own identity (Moore, 1988; Zidek, 1988).

Although Hotelling was quite vocal in his support for separate statistics departments, he was still teaching statistics in Columbia's Department of Political Science at the time of his talk at Berkeley (Reid, 1982, p. 198). After World War II, a separate Department of Statistics was created at the University of North Carolina, and Hotelling was invited to head it. Columbia did not establish a separate department to accommodate Hotelling and, in 1946, he left for North Carolina. Soon afterward, Columbia created a statistics department.

While at the University of North Carolina, Hotelling recruited professors R. C. Bose and S. N. Roy from India as well as W. Hoeffding from the Soviet Union.

Hotelling sometimes used mimeographed pages from his own treatise for teaching material, but his creation was still unfinished at the time of his death. His endeavors for perfection and his busy schedule often led to delays in the publication of his research (Levene, 1974).

He is described as being a very warmhearted, humane, considerate person who enjoyed people. During his years at Columbia and later at North Carolina, he and his second wife held open house the first Sunday of each month at his home, and all students, faculty, friends, and children were welcome. He was especially kind in assisting foreign trainees and visitors, who were often his house guests, and he was active in finding positions for European scientists displaced by the war (Levene, 1974).

Hotelling served as president of the Econometric Society during 1936–37 and of the Institute of Mathematical Statistics in 1941. He was awarded an honorary LL.D, by the University of Chicago in 1955 and an honorary D.Sc. by the University of Rochester in 1963. He was elected to the National Academy of Sciences in 1970 and to the Accademia Nazionale dei Lincei, a scholarly society of which Galileo was once a member, in 1973 (W. L. Smith, 1978).

Paul Samuelson in his 1970 Nobel Prize acceptance speech said, "Economics . . . has its heros, and the letter H that I used in my mathematical equations was not there to honor Sir William Hamilton, but rather Harold Hotelling" (W. L. Smith, 1978).

Harold Hotelling retired in 1966, suffered a stroke in 1972, and died the following year.

Jerzy Neyman (1894–1981)

The information for this brief biography of Jerzy Neyman, one of the creators of modern statistics, was selected primarily from the works of Egon Pearson (1970), Constance Reid (1982), Elizabeth Scott (1985), and Erich Lehmann (1990, 1993).

Neyman was born in 1894 in Bendery, Russia, to Polish parents. His last name was originally Splawa-Neyman, but he shortened it when he

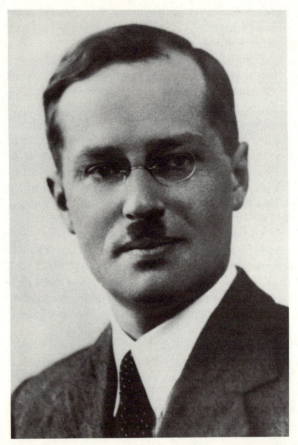

Jerzy Neyman. (From Neyman, J., *Proceedings of the Berkeley Symposium on Mathematical Statistics and Probability. Four Symposia*. Copyright © 1951–1956, Regents of the University of California. Courtesy of the University of California Press, Berkeley.)

was 30 years old. Growing up in Russia, he entered the university at Kharkov in 1912, where he was introduced to probability theory and statistics. After World War I, Poland regained its independence but soon became involved in a border war with Russia. At this time, Neyman was jailed as an enemy alien. In a 1921 prisoner exchange, the 27-year-old Neyman saw Poland for the first time.

Although Neyman admired theoretical mathematics, the statistics that he had learned in college enabled him to secure a job as a statistician at an agricultural institute. During 1921–22 he wrote several papers in which he introduced probability models to agricultural experiments, including a randomization model for a completely randomized experiment.

At the end of 1922, Neyman moved to Warsaw to assume a position at the State Meteorological Institute. However, he disliked being responsible for equipment and observations and soon found an opening as an assistant at the University of Warsaw. He lectured in mathematics and statistics, and, in 1924, obtained his doctorate from that university. It was probably at the Central Office of Statistics that he first read *Biometrika*. Student's articles were of special interest to him because the small sample experiments arose from agricultural work (Reid, 1982, p. 53).

In 1925, Neyman was granted a fellowship to study under Karl Pearson at University College, London. He believed that the mathematicians in Poland were unable to judge the importance of his statistical papers and wanted to determine whether Pearson would actually publish his work in *Biometrika* (Scott, 1985). While three of his articles concerning sample moments were published, Neyman was discontented during his year stay (1925–26) with Pearson. He found the laboratory to be old-fashioned and Pearson to be surprisingly ignorant of modern mathematics. The fact that Pearson did not understand the difference between independence and lack of correlation led to a misunderstanding that nearly terminated Neyman's stay (Lehmann, 1990).

When Neyman secured a Rockefeller fellowship for another year (1927) in the West, he decided to spend it in Paris where he once more became absorbed in his first love, pure mathematics. The stimulus that gradually prodded him back into statistics was a letter from Egon Pearson (Lehmann, 1990). Karl Pearson's son had begun to question the reasoning behind some of the recent work in statistics; his letter to Neyman began an 8-year joint effort and a lifetime correspondence.

From 1927 to 1934, Neyman worked in Poland, becoming involved in agricultural experiments, social health insurance, Polish census data, statistical research on the behavior of bacteria and viruses, and problems in the chemical industry (Scott, 1985). In 1928, he succeeded in getting a small biometric laboratory established at the Nencki Institute of Experimental Biology, and he became its first director. Funding, however, depended on the financial situation in Poland, and his meager income was a constant source of worry and stress (Lehmann, 1990; E. S. Pearson, 1970).

Neyman and Egon Pearson collaborated primarily by correspondence and several brief meetings in France and Poland as they attempted to develop general principles from which the small sample tests of Student and Fisher could be derived. In 1928, they published their fundamental two-part paper, *On the Use and Interpretation of Certain Test Criteria for Purposes of Statistical Inference*, which presented many of the basic concepts of the later Neyman–Pearson theory of hypothesis testing.

The first part of the paper considered how to determine whether it was probable that a given sample, taken as a whole, had been drawn from a specified population. To do this, the authors connected several of the most simple tests in a logical sequence and found it essential to use Fisher's principle of likelihood. They concluded that there was no single best test; instead a statistician must select a test and have a clear understanding of the process of reasoning on which the test is based. The process of reasoning is an individual matter, and the authors did not claim that the method most helpful to them would be of the greatest assistance to others. They described methods of approach.

The second part of the paper dealt with the definition of likelihood, the fundamental chi-square problem, and how to test goodness-of-fit.

In 1929, members of the ISI met in Poland. Neyman hoped that by the time of the meeting he would have saved about 50 English pounds and proposed that Egon Pearson buy him a car in London and drive to Warsaw. Pearson was astonished and many years later communicated to Constance Reid:

> He suggested that Egon Pearson, who had never driven a car, should buy one and start off in it across Europe! It was characteristic of him to make optimistic suggestions, and not to realise how he was tilting against the impossible. When rereading this letter I noted down: Here we see his intrepidity hoping to surmount all barriers in me, to carry through an impossible transaction—it

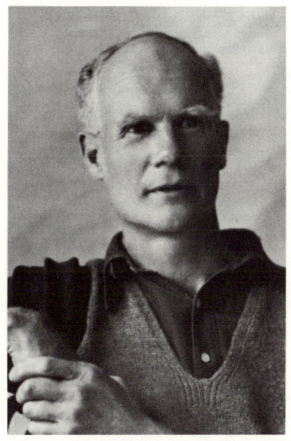

Egon S. Pearson. (Courtesy of Egon S. Pearson's daughter, Sarah Pearson.)

reminded me of that optimistic spirit, so characteristic of the Polish race, which led them 10 years later to think that they might use their cavalry against the German tanks! [Reid, 1982, p. 85]

Reid stated that nothing came of the proposal.

By 1931, the situation in Poland was becoming desperate, and Neyman wrote to Pearson:

In town I am terribly busy in getting some job for the Lab. You may have heard that we have in Poland a terrific crisis in everything. Accordingly the money from the Government given usually to the Nencki Institute will be diminished considerably and I shall have difficulties in feeding my pups [research workers in the Lab]. [E. S. Pearson, 1970]

And again in 1932:

You seem to be a little annoyed with me: in fact you have some reasons as I do not answer properly your letters. This however is really not the result of carelessness or of anything which could be offensive. I simply cannot work; the crisis and the struggle for existence takes all my time and energy. I am not sure that next year I shall not be obliged to take some job, I do not know where—in trade, perhaps, selling coal or handkerchiefs. [E. S. Pearson, 1970]

For Neyman, his continuing association with Egon Pearson was uplifting during this troubling period. They had been working on tests of statistical hypotheses since the publication of their 1928 paper and were preparing a detailed article. The issue of hypothesis testing has recurred many times in the history of statistics. Thomas Bayes is often associated with its origin because he wrote on the probability of a hypothesis based on given data, but Neyman and Pearson are given credit for establishing and developing the subject; they introduced the terms *power function* and *uniformly most powerful test*.

In their 1933 publication, *On the Problem of the Most Efficient Tests of Statistical Hypotheses*, the two men presented a new basis for choosing among criteria suitable for testing any given statistical hypothesis, H_0, with regard to an alternative hypothesis, H_1. They stated that if there are two possible criteria and if in using them there is the same chance of rejecting H_0 when it is in fact true, the choice should be that one of the two that assures the minimum chance of accepting H_0 when the true hypothesis is H_1. The best critical region assures the minimum chance of accepting H_0 when the true hypothesis is H_1. They illustrated the method for finding the best critical regions for testing both simple and composite hypotheses and, as examples, applied their method to several important problems commonly met in statistical analysis. They discussed simple and composite hypotheses, the determination of the best critical region, the test for the significance of the difference between two variances, and the test for the significance of the difference between two means.

After his father retired in 1933, Egon Pearson arranged for Neyman to return to University College, first as a senior lecturer and later as a reader (associated professor). Arriving in London in 1934, Neyman now had an assured position and a congenial working atmosphere that culminated in several keystone papers; he returned to Poland only for brief visits.

In a 1934 address (*On the Two Different Aspects of the Representative Method: The Method of Stratified Sampling and the Method of Purposive Selection*), Neyman discussed the mathematical theories underlying random sampling, stratified random sampling, and estimating the precision of the sampling. After the talk, E. S. Pearson (1934) stated:

> The particular problem considered is that of estimating certain characteristics of a heterogeneous population from a limited sample. In doing that we have to consider, if we can, how best to take a sample, how to obtain our estimate, and what measure of reliability to place on that estimate.

Pearson knew that certain assumptions were unavoidable but any assumptions must be kept to a minimum. Solving such problems required the precise mathematical analysis that Neyman had presented.

Ronald Fisher (1934) described Neyman's treatment of the subject as "luminous," and Lehmann (1990) believes that Neyman's talk and subsequent publication initiated the modern theory of survey sampling; it is probably the fundamental paper on sampling, optimal design, and confidence intervals.

The details of the Neyman–Pearson theories were quickly learned and disseminated by statisticians in all fields of research. Many efforts to construct powerful tests and others to enlarge on the presented concepts were reported (Scott, 1985). An example is the primary book on decision functions by Abraham Wald (*Statistical Decision Functions*, 1950), which is based on the Neyman–Pearson theory (Scott, 1985).

In 1970, E. S. Pearson wrote:

I think that by 1934 we had found the answers that satisfied us to most of the more tractable problems. We had now been brought up against the hard fact that mathematical models which fit the observations of the real world will not respond beyond a point to a simple theory of statistical inference. Frequency distributions so often cannot be represented by mathematical functions which yield, for example, sufficient statistics or uniformly most powerful tests!

Neyman published a third fundamental paper in 1937, *Outline of a Theory of Statistical Estimation Based on the Classical Theory of Probability*, in which he created the theory of estimation by confidence sets. He discussed the general topic of estimation, solving problems of confidence intervals, the accuracy of confidence intervals, and confidence limits.

Scott (1985) wrote:

The characteristic pattern of Neyman's research is evident in all three of these fundamental research efforts [1928, 1934, 1937] to take a rather vague statistical question and make of it a precisely stated mathematical problem for which one can search for an optimal solution. His papers established a new climate in statistical research and new directions in statistical methodology.

Neyman remained in England for 4 years during which he and Pearson established a series, *Statistical Research Memoirs*, published by University College and restricted to articles from the Department of Statistics. In 1937 Neyman was invited to give a series of lectures on sampling for the U.S. Department of Agriculture. These were published (Neyman, 1938), and an enlarged second edition (1952) includes narrations of many of his ideas. While in the United States he lectured at several universities and later that year received an unexpected letter from the chairman of the Department of Mathematics at the University of California at Berkeley offering him a position.

It may seem strange that Neyman even considered moving across the ocean to a university with no reputation in the field of statistics when he already was well situated in the statistical center of the universe. The proposal, however, appealed to him for three prevailing reasons—Berkeley had no established or formal program in statistics, and he would have free rein to develop his own theories and concepts; he realized that World War II was fast approaching, initiating fears that Poland might be destroyed, leading to his internment again as an enemy alien; and he viewed his job in England as somewhat dead-end, offering limited opportunity for advancement or for unrestrained freedom in his work (Scott, 1985; Lehmann, 1990). Neyman later said:

> In 1921 I finished my studies in Russia, and I was an alien. I came to Poland, and found myself an alien. I went to Britain, and found myself an alien. By 1938, I was feeling, all around, like a professional veteran alien. And then I came to California, and here I stopped being an alien. [Reid, 1982, p. 237]

He accepted the overseas offer and arrived in California in 1938 with his wife (from whom he later separated) and his 2-year-old son. Neyman was 44 years old, and he remained at Berkeley for the rest of his life. He liked the area and the university, and, being a good-natured and social person, he made many friends.

Over the years Berkeley became known as a prominent world center for statistics. From his Statistical Laboratory, Neyman guided the teaching program and achieved a wide student base that justified expansion of the faculty and strengthened his negotiations with the administration.

During World War II, he was heavily involved with work for the military, primarily bombing research. He studied the factors involved in dropping bombs: the aiming error, the distortion caused when the bomb is released from a moving plane, the effect of winds; in short, he learned to apply probability theory to warfare (Reid, 1982, p. 186). He made several trips to Eglin Field in Florida because he wanted closer contact with the men who actually flew the planes and dropped the bombs. He created experiments with the bomb sight trainer at Eglin to prove his new hypothesis that "the most efficient method of utilizing a given number of bombers against the same number of ships would be for several of the bombers to take on one ship instead of each bomber attacking a separate ship" (Reid, 1982, pp. 185–86).

In 1945, in celebration of the end of the conflict and the return to theoretical research, he held his first international symposium on mathematical statistics and probability. It was so successful that Neyman organized similar symposia that were held at 5-year intervals until 1970 (Lehmann, 1990).

In 1955, a separate Department of Statistics was created at Berkeley with Neyman as its chair, but he resigned the following year because he believed that the new department deserved to be led by a new and younger man (Lehmann, 1990). He continued as professor of statistics and retained directorship of the old Statistical Laboratory until his death on August 5, 1981.

Neyman's major research projects at Berkeley included "questions regarding competition of species, accident proneness, the distribution of galaxies and the expansion of the universe, the effectiveness of cloud seeding, and a model for carcinogenesis" (Lehmann, 1990).

In a 1960 article, Fisher made some disapproving remarks about Neyman's work, and Neyman replied with the *Silver Jubilee of my Dispute with Fisher* (1961). This dissension had been ongoing since 1935 and concerned primarily their approaches to hypothesis testing. Over the years, many statisticians entered the debate and expressed varying opinions. Lehmann (1993) in an unbiased analysis found areas of mutual understanding to resolve some of the two men's fundamental differences. He concluded that the theories of Fisher and Neyman are complementary rather than contradictory and that a method that combines the best features of each is possible.

Neyman has been described as an excellent teacher and a stimulating researcher who encouraged and excited his students and colleagues, cooperating with them in various projects and always doing more than his share of the work. He was considerate about acknowledging and giving credit to affiliated authors—always in exact alphabetical order (Scott, 1985). On several occasions, he spoke out for honesty and for a strict code of ethics in science (Scott, 1985).

He worked hard to maintain and support statistical organizations, arranging many meetings and conferences. He served on the council and as president of the IMS. Believing that the ISI should be opened to include academic statisticians and young researchers, he helped to form a new section, the Bernoulli Society, whose members could attend ISI sessions (Scott, 1985).

Neyman held a particular admiration for Copernicus. The 450th anniversary of the astronomer's birth was noted by Neyman in 1923 (in Poland) with a talk and the 500th anniversary in 1973 (at Berkeley) with speeches, articles, and a book, *The Heritage of Copernicus: Theories 'Pleasing to the Mind,'* edited by Neyman (Scott, 1985).

Jerzy Neyman's accomplishments were recognized internationally with many awards and medals. He was elected to the ISI, the International Astronomical Union, the U. S. National Academy of Sciences, the Swedish and Polish Academies of Science, and the Royal Society. He received the U. S. National Medal of Science and the Guy Medal in gold from the Royal Statistical Society (Scott, 1985).

More meaningful than all of the official rewards, however, was his legacy of kindness and helpfulness—he gave his warmth, talents, assistance, time, and even monetary aid to students and colleagues. He always lived beyond his means, "generously buying and spending for visitors and students out of his own pocket. Even during the war he had insisted . . . that he had to each an evening course at fifty dollars a month to get by" (Reid, 1982, p. 220). Neyman had an uncanny ability to get people to do what he wanted, often when they really did not want to do the project. He never gave up and just seemed to sweep them away with his convincing arguments. Statisticians were known to leave the room when Jerzy Neyman walked in because they knew that he would get them to do something they did not want to do (Reid, 1982, p. 267). It seems clear that, on occasion, he could be extremely stubborn. We admire him, however, because he overcame early hardships to fulfill his hopes, and his bequest to science was a wealth of publications that propelled him to acceptance as one of the great founders of modern statistics (Lehmann, 1990; Scott, 1985).

William G. Cochran (1909–1980)

When William Cochran was born in Scotland in 1909, an academic career in mathematics would have been unimaginable—most men in Rutherglen, near Glasgow, worked in smoky factories and lived in nearby tenements. However, although money was scarce, "Willie" and his older brother Oliver remembered a happy childhood playing in the neighboring woods and fields. Oliver spoke of those days at a service for Cochran at Harvard Memorial Church in 1980 (Watson, 1982).

At age 18, Willie placed first in the Glasgow University scholarship competition and was awarded funding for his college years. He was graduated in 1931 with an M.A. degree and first class honors in mathematics and natural philosophy (physics), which led to a stipend of 200 pounds yearly to attend Cambridge University for 4 years. Cochran was a mathematics student at St. John's College, Cambridge, and worked toward a Ph.D. degree in statistics (Yates, 1982). During this period, he wrote his first statistical paper, *The Distribution of Quadratic Forms in a Normal System (1934)*—the starting point for the subsequent Cochran's theorem.

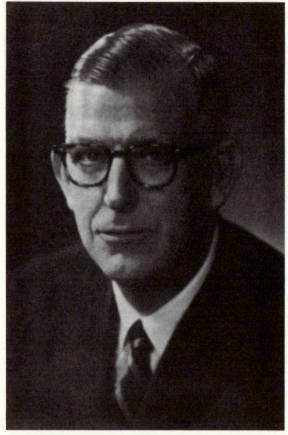

William G. Cochran. (From Watson, G. S., 1982, William Gemmell Cochran 1909–1980. *Ann Stat* **10**:1. Courtesy of the Institute of Mathematical Statistics.)

In 1934, Frank Yates asked Cochran to be his assistant at Ro-thamsted, and Cochran readily accepted even though he was obliged to stop work on his Ph.D. degree. In Great Britain at that time, jobs were scarce, and Cochran appreciated the opportunities at Rothamsted; for the next 5 years, he learned practical statistics in a research environment. During the 1920s, Ronald Fisher had succeeded in bringing researchers and statisticians together and had created new approaches to experimental design and analysis. Yates and Cochran worked closely together to further develop and apply Fisher's innovative measures to the problems of crop yields. By 1934, Rothamsted was well-known among agronomic research workers who came from all over the world to observe and learn. Cochran was exposed to experiments and problems of agriculture of diverse regions, including the tropics (Yates, 1982).

Although Fisher was the Galton Professor of Eugenics at University College, London, at this time, he remained close to the Experimental Station, and Cochran saw him frequently. Fisher also lectured at University College, and Cochran could go to London to hear him and to attend meetings of the Royal Statistical Society. Years later in a memorial tribute to Fisher, Cochran recalled that on one occasion he and Fisher were standing on a busy London street corner waiting to cross.

> Traffic was almost continuous and I was worried because Fisher could scarcely see and I would have to steer him safely across the road. Finally there was a gap, but clearly not large enough to get us across. Before I could stop him he stepped into the stream, crying over his left shoulder, "Oh, come on, Cochran. A spot of natural selection won't hurt us." [Cochran, 1967]

Cochran met his future wife Betty, an entomologist, at Ro-thamsted, and they were married in 1937 (Watson, 1982).

In 1938, he visited Ames, Iowa, and accepted a professorship offer at Iowa State College. He later withdrew his acceptance because of the impending war in Europe but, after the offer was renewed, he moved to Ames in 1939. Initially, Cochran's lack of a Ph.D. degree had caused some dismay among authorities at Ames (Yates, 1982), but Snedecor must have convinced them of Cochran's exceptional qualifications.

> During his 5 years at Rothamsted, he published some 20 papers, one-third on experimental design, one-third on sampling problems and agricultural meteorology, and the remainder on mis-cellaneous practical and theoretical problems, a creditable begin-

ning to the total of over 100 published during the whole of his career. [Yates, 1982]

Before moving to Ames, Cochran presented *Long-term Agricultural Experiments* before the Royal Statistical Society. This delivery was the high point of his years at Rothamsted, and Sir John Russell, the director of the Rothamsted Experimental Station, proposed a vote of thanks that was seconded by Ronald Fisher. Sir John reminded the audience that exactly 20 years before he had asked another young mathematician if it might be possible to get more information out of the unique long-term experiments that had been initiated at Rothamsted—wheat in 1843, barley in 1852, and marigolds in 1876. Fisher had accepted that challenge and had earned a center spotlight in statistical history.

Statistics had an unusual status at Iowa State—Snedecor had promoted Fisher's ideas, and all experimental work at the college received proper statistical consideration and treatment. Cochran lectured on sample surveys and experimental designs, and books on these subjects were published (*Experimental Designs*, with Gertrude Cox, 1950, and *Sampling Techniques*, 1953a). Ames had a close affiliation with the national Bureau of the Census because of sampling work at Iowa State, and for many years Cochran chaired an advisory panel to assist the Bureau (Watson, 1982).

In 1943, Cochran joined the Princeton Statistical Research Group directed by Samuel Wilks to work on military problems. "In 1945, he was a member of a team that surveyed the damage from Allied bombing raids to assess their efficacy" (Watson, 1982). In 1946, Gertrude Cox succeeded in recruiting Cochran to head the graduate program in experimental statistics at North Carolina State College in Raleigh. His publications during this period reflect a continuation of his earlier interests: *Design of Greenhouse Experiments for Statistical Analysis* (1946, with Cox), *Relative Accuracy of Systematic and Stratified Random Samples for a Certain Class of Populations* (1946), *Some Consequences when the Assumptions for the Analysis of Variance are not Satisfied* (1947a), and *Recent Developments in Sampling Theory in the United States* (1947b).

From 1949 to 1957, Cochran was chairman of the Department of Biostatistics in the School of Hygiene and Public Health at Johns Hopkins University, and for the first time, his work involved medical rather than agricultural problems. *Sexual Behavior in the Human Male* caused widespread consternation when it was issued in 1948, and people fought for copies. The National Research Council had supported the effort by Kinsey *et al.* and in 1950, asked the ASA to select several statisticians to evaluate the report's methodology, which was the main target of criticism. Frederick Mosteller, John Tukey, and Cochran (as chairman) were appointed by Samuel Wilks, then president of the ASA. Although Cochran's review *Satistical Problems of the Kinsey Report* (1953b) was thorough and lengthy, the ASA also issued a book that contained an expanded version of the report plus many appendices (Cochran *et al.*, 1954).

From 1954 to 1957, Cochran was involved in the triumph over poliomyelitis. The Salk vaccine had been created and produced, and the National Foundation for Infantile Paralysis selected an advisory committee, on which Cochran sat as biostatistician, to plan a trial among children. Because polio would be diagnosed in only about 50 per 100,000 people in an average year, hundreds of thousands of children would have to be enrolled. The foundation leaders told the committee that a randomized design was not to be considered because parents could not be asked to submit their children to such an experiment. A nonrandomized plan was announced—second-grade schoolchildren would be offered the new vaccine, whereas first and third graders would serve as controls. However, some state and local officials took a more scientific stand. Led by epidemiologists at the New York State Health Department, they adamantly argued that the suggested plan might result in a grave misappraisal and that a well-designed randomized double-blind study should be organized (Meier, 1984). New York officials stood firm—they would participate only if a randomized trial were offered. A compromise solution was negotiated whereby local areas were allowed to choose either the randomized or the nonrandomized method. In the final report (Francis *et al.*, 1955), about 1 million children participated in a nonrandomized trial, while 400,000 enrolled in a randomized subset. The latter group may still be the largest randomized study ever carried out (Colton, 1981). At a final press conference that was a grand public relations show on national television, members of the advisory committee sat on the platform. When each received a copy of the results, Cochran "scanned it, performed a quick mental calculation, looked up with a broad smile, and whispered to his neighbor, 'The sample size was barely large enough'" (Colton, 1981).

In the analysis of the results, the foundation's staff statisticians proposed using a Poisson model to estimate the relative effectiveness of the vaccine.

Cochran pointed out that strains of polio vary in different locales, that [the] lots of a vaccine vary in their relative effectiveness, and that for these and other reasons the assumption that the relative effectiveness of the [Salk] vaccine [was] uniform, a requirement for the Poisson analysis, was entirely untenable and the result would be a possible substantial underestimate of the standard error of the average effectiveness. [Meier, 1984]

Cochran was unable to convince the staff, and the Poisson analysis was the basis for the later claim that the vaccine had proved to be at least 60% effective in preventing polio. Subsequently, Cochran presented his analysis showing that the initially reported standard errors were too small by about 15%. It was characteristic of Cochran to make no loud protest, just as he had made no impassioned plea for randomization in the beginning. "It was Cochran's style to demonstrate and educate, not to assume the direction of activity or to do battle for one position or another" (Meier, 1984).

When a department of statistics was established at Harvard University (1957), Cochran, Mosteller, and others helped to organize it and to design the curricula.

In the early 1960s, Cochran, a heavy smoker at that time, served as the only biostatistician on the committee of the *Surgeon General's Report on Smoking and Health*. Most statisticians would not enjoy or even want to be associated with a similar study. There was no human experimental evidence to be had, no lung cancers had been produced in animals, many potential biases existed in the observational material, and prominent statisticians had declared publicly that "no reasonable conclusion adverse to cigarette smoking could be drawn from the available evidence" (Meier, 1984). However, there were many pieces of cumulative evidence relating to the harmful consequences of smoking, and these required detailed review and impartial appraisal by persons who were well aware of the possibility of bias. "Cochran was a tireless member who would not stand for loose talk or writing. He persistently warned of the limitations in interpreting the data. . . . he kept everybody honest" (Colton,1981). He was one of the authors of several editions of the Surgeon General's report (Advisory Committee to the Surgeon General, 1964), and while these summaries did not settle the issue, they allowed the federal public health establishment to take a firm stand that led to solidifying public opinion against smoking (Meier, 1984).

Cochran retired in 1976. His main contributions to statistics were in the theory and methodology of sampling surveys, the design of experiments, the analysis of variance, variance components, observational studies, and methods for strengthening chi-square tests. He was the author (or coauthor) of five books and 121 papers (Watson, 1982). He may be the only individual who served as president of the four statistical societies: the IMS in 1946–47, the ASA in 1953–54, the Biometric Society in 1954–55, and the ISI from 1976 to 1981. When gold went above $700 per ounce, Cochran joked, "Gather up my medals, now is the time to sell," for he had accumulated many: Gourock High School, 1924; Glasgow High School, 1924; McLaurin Medal for Mathematics, 1929; Cunningham Medal for Mathematics and the Isaac Newton Medal for Natural Philosophy, 1930; the Logan Medal from Glasgow University, 1931; the Guy Medal from the Royal Statistical Society, 1936; and the Wilks Medal of the ASA, 1967 (Watson, 1982).

Cochran was a very fine man, loved by all who knew him. Friends and colleagues expressed high respect for his professional life and personal principles. His intelligence, broad experience, and general knowledge made his opinions and counsel invaluable. He was also a distinguished scholar—reserved, unpretentious, candid, and extremely capable. "He was a very kind and patient teacher and generously gave his time for discussions with the students, for guiding them toward good research, for correcting their work, and for educating them to develop independent thinking" (Rao, 1984). He appeared to maintain his calm disposition, composure, and Scotsman's sense of humor even when he was ill. After suffering a stroke, he wrote to Rao in July 1979, "I have been living quietly here, and getting along fine except that my walk is still unsteady and a little drunken." Later, in September 1979, "On the way home from the Census Bureau, I apparently had a stroke which has affected my speech, writing, and balance, but not, fortunately, one-finger typing, which is why I am typing this" (Rao, 1984). He died on March 29, 1980.

CHAPTER 5

Clinical Trials in the United States

Randomization was used in many types of agricultural, industrial, laboratory, and animal experiments before it was applied to medical trials in the 1950s, and its superiority over selected treatment assignments was undisputed.

In 1951, the National Heart Institute (NHI), now known as the National Heart, Lung and Blood Institute, took part in its first multicenter randomized clinical trial, which related to rheumatic fever and rheumatic heart disease (Rheumatic Fever Working Party, 1960). The trial involved 497 children under the age of 16 who were enrolled in 12 centers in the United Kingdom, the United States, and Canada. The investigators compared ACTH, cortisone, and aspirin in the treatment of rheumatic fever and the prevention of rheumatic heart disease. They found no differences in the efficacy of the three drugs; the status of the heart at the start of treatment was the major factor related to outcome. Except for an NHI statistician who served as a consultant, the NHI had no scientific involvement in the trial and did not participate in another randomized trial until the 1960s (Halperin *et al.*, 1990).

In 1954, members of Congress asked officials at the National Cancer Institute (NCI) to organize a comprehensive program for research in cancer chemotherapy, and Congress awarded almost $1 million in grants to a few prominent research institutions and medical schools to get the mission started (Sessoms, 1960). In 1955, the Cancer Chemotherapy National Service Center (CCNSC) was established to coordinate and operate the entire research enterprise through programs for testing a large number of new compounds in tissue culture and animal systems (mainly mice) and organizing cooperative clinical trials of the most effective agents. In the early randomized trials, investigators studied various types of cancer and usually conducted a comparison of chemotherapeutic regimens. Money was available for these endeavors because of the congressional funding.

At that time, critics expressed the viewpoint that essentially random searches for effective chemotherapeutic agents were futile and "as much energy was expended in the scientific community to stop cancer drug development as was exerted to get it off the ground" (DeVita, 1984). Cancer had always been considered a localized disease that was amenable to surgery or radiation if diagnosed early. The medical community was very slow to view it as a systemic illness; physicians had to be convinced, over time, to accept chemotherapy. Today, we realize that often cancer is a systemic disease almost from the onset, with clinically unrecognized micrometastases (Zubrod, 1979).

Cancer Clinical Trials Groups

During the late 1950s, the clinical panel of the CCNSC supervised the organization of cooperative groups to conduct clinical trials in cancer. C. Gordon Zubrod, clinical director of the NCI, was primarily responsible for organizing the groups, while Marvin Schneiderman, a biostatistician, recruited the statisticians and statistical centers (Gehan and Schneiderman, 1990). Through the leadership of Zubrod, who was strongly influenced by a 1955 article by Louis Lasagna on conducting clinical trials, it was recognized from the beginning that it was important to have a clinician to lead each cooperative group and to have a statistical center involved in the design, randomization of patients, and analysis and interpretation of data.

During the first few years, seven groups were established: Acute Leukemia Groups A and B; the Eastern, Southeastern, Western, and Southwestern groups; and the University group for prostate studies. By 1960, there were 11 cooperative clinical study groups, each comprising a number of universities and/or Veterans Administration hospitals, medical centers, and a statistical coordinating center (Cancer Chemotherapy National Service Center, 1960). "The present structure of the Cooperative Groups has resulted from attrition, reorganization, and consolidation" (Zelen et al., 1980).

The first randomized clinical trial at the NCI was planned in 1954, begun in 1955, and results published in 1958 (Frei *et al.*, 1958) (see Chapter 6 for details). From the beginning, there was acceptance of the principles of the randomization of patients and the statistical analysis of data. The early trials conducted in the cooperative groups program were nearly all prospective randomized clinical trials, and this became accepted as the primary method for the comparative evaluation of therapies. As the cooperative groups program evolved, each new drug progressed through a series of clinical trials: phase I to determine dosage, phase II to determine preliminary efficacy, and phase III to compare the effectiveness of treatments.

Statistical methodological developments to analyze data from clinical trials were introduced by the mid-1960s. These included a plan for phase II trials (Gehan, 1961); a generalization of the Wilcoxon test to compare survival distributions with right-censored data (Gehan, 1965); a test of proportional hazards for comparing two survival distributions, which was a generalization of the Mantel–Haenszel test (Mantel and Haenszel, 1959) to survival distribution applications (Mantel, 1966); and an exponential regression model relating survival time to explanatory variables (Feigl and Zelen, 1965). Thus, from the beginning, the prospective randomized clinical trial was the cornerstone for the comparative evaluation of therapies in the cooperative groups clinical trials program.

Congressional allocations increased; in 1970, the NCI's budget was $180 million, and by 1977, it had reached $815 million (Schmidt, 1977). According to Shorter, "Congress thought it was financing revolutionary cancer therapies. What it did was to help finance with cancer money the revolution in biotechnology. For one thing, about half of the cancer institute's budget would be spent on basic research rather than on applied studies" (Shorter, 1987). Out of this research came most of the biochemistry of recombinant DNA technology (Shorter, 1987). However, a mature clinical trials program for the evaluation of various types of cancer therapies, including chemotherapy, surgery, radiotherapy, and bone marrow transplantation, also developed from the early research at the NCI.

By the early 1970s, computers began to take over substantial and important functions in the data management, not only at the large statistical centers but for every statistician worldwide. Today, many analyses entail calculations that are too time consuming without computer capability.

Randomized versus Historical Control Studies

Background

Let us take out of the hospitals, out of the Camps, or from else-where, 200, or 500 poor People, that have Fevers, Pleurisies, & c. Let us divide them into halfes, let us cast lots, that one half of them may fall to my share, and the other to yours; . . . we shall see how many funerals both of us shall have: But let the reward of the contention or wager, be 300 florens, deposited on both sides. [van Helmont, 1662, quoted in Armitage, 1982]

The casting of lots can be considered as randomization of an earlier era. It fixed the responsibility for choosing the groups on chance, not on the participating physicians. Investigators today, however, do not usually set wagers on the outcomes.

Patients who agree to cooperate in a clinical trial, whether randomized or not, tend to get more attention and better care than nonparticipants. Painstaking consideration has gone into every aspect of the protocol with both treatment and control groups benefiting from excellent supportive measures. Diagnostic studies are thorough, and there is close observation of patients during follow-up, with visits scheduled at regular intervals. All this, plus medication, is supplied at no cost to the patient. Each year more than 500,000 Americans agree to be test subjects in clinical trials (Berkman, 1991).

Recently, however, the cost of clinical trials, especially those involving expensive regimens such as bone marrow transplantation, has come under close scrutiny by funding agencies and medical insurance companies, making it more tenuous to find firm support for clinical trials research.

Some physicians are reluctant to participate in cooperative randomized trials because, often, they are given no author listing or credit in the published reports, even though they contribute much time and effort to the projects. Most clinicians who participate in large cancer studies have little or no input into the protocol; their task is to recruit patients and to treat them precisely as dictated by the procedural manual.

The bureaucracy of the cancer clinical trials study groups has become large and cumbersome, and, once the gears are turning, trials tend to progress methodically step by step according to the original plan. Such a system tends to restrain clinical investigators from generating original ideas or inventive solutions to problems. Some investigators, therefore, prefer to organize and publish their own small-scale studies of 50 to 100 patients, leaving the larger randomized studies to cooperative groups. Peto and Easton (1989) wrote that "the major difficulty in achieving large patient entry to randomized studies is the reluctance of many oncologists to participate in collaborative clinical research."

These authors also believe that the protocols of some randomized trials include pointless criteria that make exacting demands on busy clinicians, and such requirements curb their participation. The inconvenience of stringent eligibility stipulations, special investigations, diagnostic review, detailed documentation of treatment, and frequent follow-ups may far outweigh any benefit. Lengthy elaborations of treatment are impossible to analyze in relation to outcome. Essentially, Peto and Easton argue for large clinical trials, with the assumption that there is likely to be only a small difference in therapeutic outcomes between randomized therapies, making large trials necessary to establish that small advances in prognosis are real. With this approach, one is basically comparing two strategies for the administration of treatment. Extensive evaluation of each component of the treatment program is not vital for proving the superiority of a program if the number of patients is large.

Funding

A large multicenter cancer clinical trial may involve many principal investigators for a period of 5 to 10 years. In 1990, there were ten major cooperative clinical trial groups sponsored by the NCI that involved more than 4600 clinical investigators who were conducting approximately 400 protocol studies in more than 23,000 patients with cancer (Gehan, 1991). The total cost of the NCI cooperative clinical trials program in 1990 was $60,208,000.

Funding is easier to obtain for randomized trials than for historical control studies. The former is the standard for evaluating the relative efficacy of therapies within the cooperative group clinical trials program, and it is more difficult to persuade review committees to provide funding for nonrandomized studies.

Assignment of Patients to Treatment

The superiority of randomization over other methods of choosing or determining patients for treatment and control groups lies foremost in the elimination of selection bias that may derive from the investigator. The two groups must be suitable for comparison at the beginning, during, and at the end of the study. Adherence to a proper randomization scheme removes the possibility of physician influence in assigning patients to a treatment or control group. Ideally, any difference in the outcomes between the two groups will be caused solely by the treatment being tested. If it is later determined that there were differences in relevant characteristics or that partiality existed when the groups were set up, the usefulness and worth of the study is jeopardized.

In clinical trials, it is especially perilous to eliminate persons from the analysis because they are atypical, inadequately treated, or inevaluable. The allocated treatment is often discontinued in patients with cancer because they are too ill, they are not responding to the therapy, or they experience dangerous toxic effects. Although they have a poor prognosis, if these people are not included, the remaining group will exhibit a false improved survival rate regardless of the influence of the treatment being tested (Peto and Easton, 1989). Removing a small scattering of patients will have a minimal effect in a large trial, but it can carry a drastic weight in a small study. The randomization scheme eliminates this pitfall if statisticians include every person allocated to a regimen whether or not that regimen is carried out. With historical controls, it may be difficult or impossible to identify and recover records on all eligible patients who presented at the earlier time period (Peto and Easton, 1989).

Before beginning any calculations on the results of a trial, the statistician must determine whether the treatment groups can be compared and whether the groups are truly representative of the population suffering from the illness being studied. If disparity exists, comparison of therapeutic regimens should be carried out in comparable subgroups or a model should be used to adjust for the imbalance in prognostic features.

Although some authors state that statisticians can adjust for selection bias, Byar (1991) has cautioned that, at best, "adjustment procedures are only partially effective in removing biases," and that "doubts always remain."

On the other hand, in contrast to historical control trials, randomized clinical trials require more patients and, therefore, more recruiting time to achieve the desired number of participants. When comparing a new treatment with a standard treatment, the use of a historical control group (with an established response rate) requires a sample size one-fourth that needed for a randomized control study of the same statistical significance and power specification (Gehan and Freireich, 1974). This would translate into about a 75% reduction in the number of months required for the historically controlled trial, assuming that patients have been recruited at a given rate per month. The savings in the number of patients derives from the assumption that the response rate in the historical control group is known.

In some situations, as in studying a rare disease, only a small number of patients will be obtainable, and a randomized trial may not be a realistic choice. Also, surgeons have expressed opposition to randomization in some types of surgical trials and question its suitability in trials evaluating new operations (van der Linden, 1980; Bonchek, 1979). The government has supplied financial support for early randomized trials of various new surgical procedures, but some studies have been unproductive because techniques were refined and changed and trials were invalidated before they were completed. "Abandonment of a flawed or obsolete randomized study involves an admission of error and a loss of financial support—a form of academic suicide" (Bonchek, 1979).

Most investigators believe that a trial design should be selected only after studying all facets of the question to be answered. Statisticians have emphasized the requirement that studies must be large enough to have a high probability (i.e., statistical power) of detecting a clinically significant difference between treatments. Investigators, however, tend to overestimate patient recruitment, and some projects are forced to close with fewer than the desired number of admissions. This can present a problem in both randomized and historical control studies, but it is a lesser concern for the latter because there is no need to accrue patients for a control group.

In recent years, as people have become more knowledgeable about choices in cancer therapy and more cognizant of the randomization process, some investigators have experienced difficulty in recruiting patients for randomized clinical trials.

In 1984, Gehan reported that a Mayo Clinic study of surgery alone versus surgery plus adjuvant chemotherapy in patients with osteosarcoma was impaired because only 38 of the 110 eligible patients accepted randomization. This was primarily because some physicians and patients were aware that adjuvant chemotherapy had been demonstrated to be more effective than no adjuvant chemotherapy in well-conducted nonrandomized studies (Sutow et al., 1978).

It is difficult to conduct a randomized study and to obtain informed consent from patients when radically different types of therapy are being compared. For example, the Southwest Oncology Group spent 3 years planning the design of a study on radiotherapy versus radical surgery in patients with localized prostate cancer, stage B (Gehan, 1984). The major difficulty the group had was getting physicians to agree to assign patients by random allocation to such radically different treatments.

To resolve this type of problem, Zelen proposed a "randomized consent design" (Zelen, 1979). In his design, a patient is randomly assigned to one of two groups: "do not seek consent" (in which the person receives the control or standard treatment) or "seek consent" (in which the person is asked to accept the experimental treatment). If P is the proportion of patients accepting the experimental treatment, then the efficiency of this design relative to a conventional randomized study is P^2. This design, in itself, however, is controversial because patients would be participating in a randomized clinical trial without their knowledge of the true situation (Fost, 1979).

A West German breast preservation trial of "small cancer" was started in 1983 using a modified Zelen design. When primary tumor excision and axillary dissection had proved the existence of a small localized malignancy, informed consent was sought. The patient then decided whether to accept or reject randomization. This process produced three groups of patients in the trial: those who accepted randomization, those who chose standard mastectomy, and those who chose breast-preserving radiotherapy. Of the first 650 patients recruited from 66 participating centers, only 10% agreed to accept randomization, whereas 30% preferred mastectomy, and 60% chose radiotherapy (Olschewski et al., 1988).

Comparability of Patient Groups

Randomization helps to create equable or balanced groups, not only for factors that contribute to the prognosis in the illness being studied, but also for other demographic or relevant data in the patients' medical histories. This information usually appears in the final report of a clinical trial under "Comparability of patient groups" and describes the extent of the balance or imbalance between the treated and control groups. Of course, adjustment for imbalance in baseline variables can be undertaken only when the important prognostic variables are known. Statisticians can simultaneously evaluate all of the variables that affect major endpoints, and thus make it easier to detect real differences (Zelen et al., 1980).

Randomization is considered to be the best way to facilitate the equalization of various factors between groups, whether the factors are generally recognized or are unsuspected. Disparity will appear more often in small trials; large numbers of patients tend to even out or limit disproportionality.

Procedures for statistical adjustment, such as regression models, are used by both randomizers and nonrandomizers to make treatment comparisons that include considering the prognostic characteristics of the patients (Freireich and Gehan, 1979). Discussing historical controls, Armitage (1982) wrote:

> Adjustments for baseline differences may well allow properly for discrepancies in the chosen variables, but they provide no safeguard against possible disparities in other respects. Not only may the comparisons be biased, but there is no way of measuring the extent of the bias.

Patients may be stratified (in either randomized or historical control trials) according to the values of known prognostic characteristics. The statistician for a randomized study randomly assigns patients within each stratum and usually allots equal numbers of patients to each treatment within the stratum. This provides an approximately equivalent number of patients on each treatment at the close of the trial. In a historical control study, patients enter strata depending on the order in which they show up for treatment, and there must be a sufficiently large historical control group to assure a balance of treated and control patients within each stratum.

All statisticians, however, are very limited in the number of prognostic variables that can be used for stratification. In cancer, the known prognostic variables may be numerous. In breast cancer, for example, factors known to influence prognosis include stage of disease, menopausal status, size of tumor, and number of positive nodes. If one

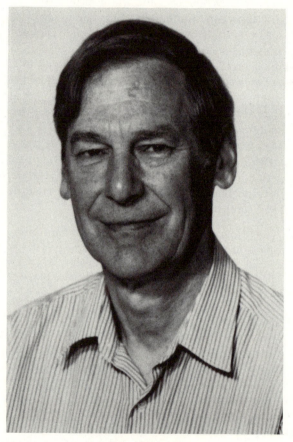

Peter Armitage.

assumes two possibilities for each factor, this leads to a total of $2 \times 2 \times 2 \times 2 = 16$ strata. As the number of prognostic variables increases, the number of strata goes up by a multiplicative factor rather than an additive factor. Usually, it is not feasible to stratify patients into more than eight strata because the number of patients in each stratum will be too small.

Also, one should include only variables strongly related to prognosis and not strongly related to each other. For example, age and menopausal status would not be meaningful as two variables.

Missing Information

A randomized study with an explicit protocol and rules for checking all documents should have no missing data at the time of analysis. Investigators using historical control groups may find that certain observations or tests, such as progesterone status for breast cancer or certain biological marker studies, may simply not have been done for patients in the historical control group. In a prospective randomized study, baseline data would be obtained for both treatment and control groups.

In a succession of cancer trials, however, patients from the last trial are frequently used as a control group for the new study. This historical control group would have been treated recently so that patient characteristics, diagnostic criteria, supportive therapy, and even medical personnel have probably not changed. If a change were made, as in definition of endpoint, this would be recognized, and the endpoints of the historical group could be redefined.

The clinical cooperative cancer centers groups, which proceed methodically from one study to the next, are directed by experienced principal investigators, and historical controls have been practicable in many instances. With such established procedures, and with computer files on past patients, there is less likelihood of missing information.

Changes with Time

Changes in patient populations, diagnostic methods, or supportive care will not enter into a prospective randomized study because patients are admitted concurrently to treatment or control groups, and any change that occurs during the course of the study will affect treatment and control cohorts alike. This is an advantage for randomization.

In a historical control cancer study, the primary investigator would certainly be aware of any significant change that might have taken place since the control study was completed. If new diagnostic methods have been instituted, if staging procedures or nomenclature have been updated, if some supportive measure has become more widely available, or if a better dosage schedule for administering a chemotherapeutic agent has reduced adverse effects, these factors would be known.

Taking the extensive research accomplished on prognostic factors in all types of cancers into account, it seems highly unlikely that some mystery variable (strongly related to outcome after having accounted for known prognostic factors) is going to be distributed disproportionately between treated and historical control groups. If several prognostic factors have been used in matching treated and historical control groups, it is reasonable to expect that an unknown prognostic factor would account for less of the remaining random variation than had already been accounted for by known factors.

Whether to undertake a historical control study depends on more important factors, such as ethics, availability of patients, and expected treatment differences, than on whether one should try to account for an unknown prognostic variable.

Validity of Tests of Statistical Significance

The statistician who reports the results of a randomized clinical trial has the assurance that his significance tests are valid. This advantage stems mainly from statistical theory because the randomization process makes it possible to ascribe a probability distribution to the difference in results between treatment groups receiving identically effective therapies and to assign significance levels to the observed differences. In other words, the statistical significance level achieved can be ascertained from the information gathered in the trial (Byar *et al.*, 1976).

With historically controlled trials, the statistician must assume that the differences in the characteristics of the patients between the earlier time period (historical control group) and the later time period (assigned treatment group) are effectively equivalent to those that would arise if the patients were sampled from a single population and then randomly assigned to treated or control groups (Gehan, 1984).

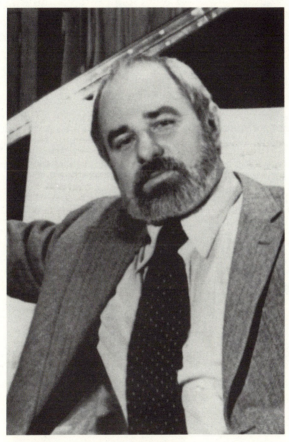

David P. Byar. (Courtesy of Dorothy L. Dowty, Biometry Branch, National Institutes of Health, Department of Health and Human Services.)

Providing Clear Answers

Neither randomized nor nonrandomized studies always provide unqualified, explicit answers. Sometimes, flaws in the management of a study can be pinpointed, but often it appears that investigators complied correctly with all of the standard procedures. Byar *et al.* (1976) wrote that discordant results among nonrandomized trials had frequently led to confusion and had stimulated the selection of a randomized trial as a more scientific choice.

The principal investigators in the University Working Group Diabetes Project discontinued the use of tolbutamide before the end of the large, cooperative randomized clinical trial because of an unexpected disproportionate number of cardiovascular deaths in the tolbutamide-treated group (University Working Group Diabetes Program, 1970). Practicing physicians, however, have not been deterred by this and have continued to prescribe tolbutamide. Whether this drug contributes to cardiovascular problems remains undetermined.

The disclosure that only 26% of all of the patients in that trial had maintained their initially assigned treatment for the total follow-up period (Feinstein, 1976; Committee for the Assessment of Biometric Aspects of Controlled Trials of Hypoglycemic Agents, 1975) was startling to readers and must have been disconcerting for the clinicians and statisticians involved. Practicing physicians did not believe that the final analysis was credible or reliable when there were so many transfers from one treatment to another. Critics also stated that practicing physicians would not have managed their diabetic patients as the protocol required. Modification of the dosage of assigned drugs was not permitted (except in the flexible insulin group) on the basis of blood glucose levels alone. Alterations were allowed only if the patient "could not be safely maintained on the assigned medication schedule" (Committee for the Assessment of Biometric Aspects of Controlled Trials of Hypoglycemic Agents, 1975).

> . . . a clinical trial of therapy must be designed as a *clinical* trial of therapy. If standards of clinical sensibility and scientific validity are sacrificed for standards of statistical theory and computer compatibility, the mortally wounded data cannot be salvaged by extensive efforts in mathematical rehabilitation. The results will remain uninterpretable in clinical practice and unacceptable in clinical science. [Feinstein, 1976]

Social Merit

"Although randomized clinical trials are very complex, expensive, and time-consuming experiments, they remain the most useful tool for comparisons of treatments" (Byar et al., 1976).

For biomedical research, the authors of ethical models, such as the Declaration of Helsinki and the Nuremberg Code, have emphasized that research must be warranted and should have value for society. "Moreover, there is a general consensus that research cannot be justified ethically unless it is designed sufficiently well that there is a reasonable expectation that it will accomplish its purpose" (Levine, 1991).

Because randomized trials are generally believed to be the most effective means, they are regarded as the most likely to accomplish the purpose stated in the protocol. Members of the institutional review boards and the National Institutes of Health or NCI study sections might judge such trials with a more favorable or approving attitude (Levine, 1991).

> The [federal] government has been involved for some years in requiring randomized clinical trials of drugs as part of a regulatory process. . . . The randomized clinical trial can only become more important as a basis for government health policy decisions. [Banta, 1982]

The Physician/Patient Relationship

"In the assessment of a treatment, medicine always has proceeded, and always must proceed, by way of experiment" (Hill, 1963). The experiment may be simply prescribing a treatment for a patient or group of patients and observing and recording the results. Nevertheless, this is human experimentation, and the physician should treat patients in such a way as to gain the maximum information about the patients and the disease. Ultimately, it may be necessary to undertake a randomized clinical trial or a historical control study. "Any belief that the controlled trial is the only way would mean not that the pendulum had swung too far but that it had come right off its hook" (Hill, 1966).

Physicians who participate in clinical trials must explain the research plan and the informed consent document to the patient and must give adequate consideration to the risk/benefit ratio and to safety (Rosner, 1987). The ethical dilemma of the randomized trial has been under consideration since the early 1960s, and the discussion has sometimes become heated in recent years.

Hill (1963) listed six ethical issues that should be considered and solved before a trial is begun. Atkins (1966) reduced this number to one: "If we would allow a member of our own family to enter the trial, it is ethical; if not, it is not ethical."

If a physician participating in a randomized study believes that no treatment being tested is preferred, and he would have no predisposition to select one treatment over the other for a member of his own family, he would face no ethical dilemma (clinical equipoise). This situation, however, must be very infrequent.

Physicians discussing a randomized trial with patients would ordinarily have had experience with the therapy of the disease under study and would almost surely have some opinions and preferences. When a new therapy for cancer is ready for a randomized trial, a great deal of information has already been disseminated. For a clinician to consider the advantages and disadvantages of both treatments to be equal must be highly unusual. Yet, ethically, he should subscribe to this belief.

Some authors have argued that even though a physician may have a preference, the fact that neither treatment has been proved to be superior is ample ethical justification for his participation in a random allocation trial. This argument may carry little weight, however, when well-conducted pilot or historical control studies have established the superiority of a particular treatment. A good example is the nonrandomized trial of MOPP (Mustargen, Oncovin, procarbazine, and prednisone) in advanced Hodgkin's disease. MOPP quadrupled the complete remission rate to 81% and prolonged relapse-free survival (DeVita *et al.*, 1970). After publication of that report, one would assume that very few patients would enter a randomized study in view of the possibility of not receiving MOPP. Surprisingly, 5 years later a randomized clinical trial was reported; 61 patients with advanced Hodgkin's disease were treated with MOPP, while 47 were treated with nitrogen mustard alone. The authors wanted to "determine whether the improved therapeutic effectiveness of combination chemotherapy was due to the use of a combination of drugs or might be achieved with a single agent if given as intensively and for as long a period" (Huguley *et al.*, 1975). Their complete remission rate of 47.5% with MOPP was significantly better than the 12.8% with nitrogen mustard ($p < 0.05$); remissions lasted longer and survival was significantly better with MOPP.

Generally, if an established standard therapy is already in place, the trial organizers would be testing a new treatment only if they, as experts in the field, believed that it offered the possibility of superior results without undue toxic effects. For many types of cancer, the standard treatment is very unsatisfactory, leading to a constant search for better therapies, with numerous chemotherapeutic agents being introduced. If one of these drugs appears to be particularly promising by preliminary experiments, and a randomized trial is under consideration, should half of the participating patients be randomly allocated to receive a known poor treatment and half allocated to the new product offering hope of a better result? Would a clinical physician be acting in the best interest of the patient by recommending that the person enter the trial?

Patients with cancer are frequently willing to risk the severe toxic effects that may occur with an unproved agent, and, sometimes, the drug is not available to them unless they agree to become a subject in a randomized trial. The situation is especially distressing when a patient travels to a large cancer center expecting to receive the latest innovative therapy and is greeted with the news that he must submit to randomization with only a 50% chance of receiving the desired treatment. "Patients participating in a clinical research program should have the opportunity to be the primary beneficiaries of that research" (Freireich and Gehan, 1979). The individual patient with cancer should receive the new experimental therapy if he so desires and should not have to submit to randomization for the benefit of future sufferers.

What course should be followed if, while a randomized study is in process, one treatment appears to be superior? Should new admissions be recruited? Should the entire procedure come to a halt, thus forsaking the knowledge to be gained by a completed trial as planned? Some clinicians believe that, on ethical grounds, they should not be obliged to continue giving a patient a supposedly inferior therapy. Should all patients be switched to the favored medication, even those doing well on the apparently inferior one? Would continuation of the trial in order to obtain a definite, clear result be the most ethical choice in the long-term consideration?

To circumvent some of these problems, statisticians have developed techniques for sequentially controlled clinical trials (see Chapter 6). During the trial, interim analyses are carried out, and if the difference in efficacy between the treatments exceeds limits that have been prespecified in the planning stage, the trial is stopped and the conclusions reported at valid statistical significance levels.

Today, all institutes of the NIH, including the NCI, frequently use an independent Data Monitoring Committee (DMC) to oversee a randomized clinical trial. The committee consists of clinicians, statisticians, and others who are not associated with the group conducting the trial. It reviews the data at regular intervals for differences in outcomes between treatments and for toxic side effects; it considers changes in design or termination of the study based on results accumulated. Participating investigators are not informed of the current comparisons between therapies, and therefore are not prejudiced and can continue to enter their patients in an ethical manner. They essentially delegate their responsibility to the DMC (Fleming, 1992).

Discussions of the ethical responsibilities of physicians have involved debates about whether the interest of the individual patients should be sacrificed for the potential benefit of future patients (the obligation of social beneficence). Should all lives, present or future, be considered equally valuable? Hellman and Hellman (1991) say

> Even if randomized clinical trials were much better than any alternative, the ethical dilemmas they present may put their use at variance with the primary obligations of the physician. In this regard, Angell [1984] cautions, "If this commitment to the patient is attenuated, even for so good a cause as benefits to future patients, the implicit assumptions of the doctor/patient relationship are violated."
>
> The risk of such attenuation by the randomized trial is great. The AIDS activists have brought this dramatically to the attention of the academic medical community. . . . We must develop and use alternative methods for acquiring clinical knowledge.

The randomized trial may tend to promote an adversarial feeling between physician and patient. As discussed by Eberbach (1987), the patient is interested in his own life and survival and wants a treatment designed for his specific disease and overall circumstances. He is not enthusiastic about his course of therapy being left to chance. Contrarily, the clinical investigator wants his trial to be valid and successful—not weakened by any deviation from the protocol that might diminish the value of the data. The tension between these viewpoints tends to degrade the physician/patient relationship.

Also, the impersonal technique of randomization may give the physician a sense of isolation from any guilt for the patient's bad luck of receiving an inferior treatment. Along this same line, Foster Lindley, a professor of philosophy, has written that the practice of randomization existed in biblical times as a means of avoiding responsibility for making important choices.

Lots were cast, thus transferring the responsibility for the selection to God.

> The physician may randomize for many reasons, but by doing so, she is able to effect a state of mind whereby she has no sense of responsibility to a patient for a given allocation. . . . The moral issue raised by the parallel trial can be, with randomization, anesthesized as the less fortunate patient is selected not by the investigator, but by chance. [Lindley, 1991]

Hill (1987) wrote, "It is perhaps widely believed that randomization per se contributes to the ethical problem inherent in a clinical trial. In my view it plays no such part." He regarded randomization as merely a technique for producing two groups in an unbiased way and securing, as far as possible, their comparability.

The substance of the ethical problem was condensed by Verstraete (1979) who wrote that ". . . the happiness of statisticians with great numbers is not always easily reconciled to the clinician's view of offering the best for each individual patient—the dilemma between medical science and humanism."

Convincing the Medical Community

In recent years and for many reasons, physicians have tended to reject results obtained in nonrandomized patient trials and to show confidence in the outcomes of randomized ones.

Looking back, however, the public has been willing to trust a physician's personal experience, and, in many instances, physicians have accepted the results of nonrandomized trials if they were well designed and conducted. They have even adopted therapies described by anecdotal case reports. In the early days of cancer chemotherapy, physicians accepted such claims of success with a small group of patients because there was no known beneficial treatment, and clinical physicians were eager and anxious to try any possibility.

Outstanding examples are the report by Farber et al. (1948), which described the use of a folic acid antagonist to prolong temporary remissions in 10 of 16 children with acute leukemia, and the studies of

Greenspan *et al.* in the early 1960s, which advocated combination chemotherapy for advanced breast cancer. The latter authors reported on treating 40 women suffering from resistant or recurrent advanced metastatic disease with simultaneous doses of methotrexate and thio-TEPA (Greenspan *et al.*, 1963). They were the first to use two agents together in the treatment of metastatic breast carcinoma, reporting responses in 60 to 80% of patients (Smalley *et al.*, 1976). "As recently as 1960, the authoritative text of Pack and Ariel failed to mention cytotoxic chemotherapy as an accepted modality of treatment for the advanced metastatic patient" (Greenspan *et al.*, 1963).

The pioneer study by Greenspan *et al.* was very important because combination chemotherapy became the accepted treatment for metastatic, locally advanced, or relapsed breast cancer. Later, Goldenberg *et al.* (1973) in a randomized study confirmed the superiority of combination over single-agent chemotherapy in advanced breast cancer, although they used different drugs than Greenspan *et al.*

Today, practicing physicians give more credence to randomized clinical trials and tend to use knowledge of the results in making decisions. Sometimes, after an uncontrolled pilot study has been done to test a new anticancer agent, researchers will agree that results should be confirmed by a randomized trial, but this has not always been forthcoming. Also, the situation may be one in which patients are randomly allocated to an apparently better new therapy versus a control therapy that has had rather poor results.

Some antineoplastic agents have been used on hundreds of patients without acceptable comparative studies with other agents to ascertain relative efficacy and toxic effects. L-Asparaginase, mithramycin, and estrogen (for carcinoma of the prostate) have been cited as outstanding examples of this failing.

Historically, new therapies have always been subjected to confirmation, and ultimately, to be accepted, their value must be substantiated by many physicians working under variable conditions with different patients. A question, however, is whether the confirmation study needs to be a randomized control study or whether studying the new therapy in a large group of patients would be sufficient. While physicians tend to accept the results of randomized studies, they are also impressed by new therapies that demonstrate substantial evidence of improvement over a standard therapy. In this circumstance, clinicians should at least be convinced to undertake a confirmation study.

Advances in Cancer Therapy

Historically, several important concepts in cancer medicine were established by early randomized trials. Independent action of the chemotherapeutic drugs 6-mercaptopurine and methotrexate was demonstrated for the first time by Frei *et al.* (1961), in a study that also provided the first conclusive evidence that combination chemotherapy could improve the complete remission rate in patients with acute leukemia.

The value of treating patients who have acute leukemia while they are in a disease-free state was established in a randomized trial by Freireich *et al.* (1963). This study showed that the action and usefulness of an agent could be proved by its ability to prolong remission in contrast to its activity for inducing remission.

Other pioneering randomized trials involving patients with leukemia indicated that it was not necessary to reduce the dosage when certain chemotherapy drugs were used in combination; each drug could be administered at an optimum (or nearly optimum) dosage without undue hazard to the patient if the types of toxic effects for each drug were different (nonoverlapping toxicity).

On the other hand, the list of important therapeutic advances in patients with cancer is more impressive for nonrandomized studies. Both before and since the publication of the first randomized cancer trial (1958), many chemotherapeutic agents were discovered, evaluated, and administered without prospective clinical trials involving the random allocation of patients. A partial list of these drugs includes nitrogen mustard, methotrexate, 6-mercaptopurine, thioguanine, prednisone, L-asparaginase, vincristine (Oncovin), arabinosylcytosine (Ara-C), and doxorubicin (Adriamycin).

All of these agents have subsequently been tested in randomized trials, either alone or as components of combination regimens. However, only in unusual circumstances is a single trial totally convincing (Byar, 1991).

A study using historical controls can supply good evidence of essential differences in treatment outcomes if the historical patients have the same span of disease severity as the present group of patients (Peto and Easton, 1989). Trials involving patients with childhood leukemia by the British Medical Research Council included almost all cases diagnosed in a particular area regardless of presenting characteristics. "Even comparisons between results of childhood acute lymphoblastic leukemia treatment in different countries appear to be reasonably reliable and have contributed more to improvements in treatment than the results of randomized trials" (Peto *et al.*, 1986).

Legal Requirements

At the present time, investigators using humans in research must review legal stipulations as well as ethical considerations. Written, signed, informed consent must be obtained from all patients in a clinical trial, and participants must be aware of their right to withdraw from the study at any time. The trial must be monitored throughout its duration with respect to truthfulness, confidentiality, fidelity, and the individual's dignity and privacy (Villeneuve, 1990).

A survey of 170 oncologists from eight countries (Taylor and Kelner, 1987) revealed that physicians regarded informed consent as an intrusion into the physician/patient relationship. The constraints of procuring consent weakened their interest in participating in research projects. Taylor and Kelner believe that legal restrictions associated with the introduction of new technologies critically affect the practice of medicine.

In addition to informed consent, certain types of clinical trials are regulated by existing legal controls. For example, studies of human gene therapy must follow the federal Guidelines for Research Involving Recombinant DNA Molecules (Areen and King, 1990), and the NIH has an Office for Protection from Research Risks.

Judicial oversight may become a significant mechanism for regulation of clinical trials. Patients may have legal recourse if the consequences of a study affect them unfavorably in any way. Lawyers have become very aware of the ethics of clinical trials and of patients' rights (Brown, 1970); the vocal AIDS activist groups have forced these issues into the headlines. Not only have they lobbied for faster processing of new therapies by the Food and Drug Administration, but some protesters want promising new drugs to be made available to all people with AIDS and to those who are HIV-positive.

Byar (1991) mentions the difficulties faced by 21 experienced statisticians who were considering design issues for trials involving people with AIDS. "We agreed to a set of criteria that should be considered when deciding whether an uncontrolled phase III trial of a new therapy could be justified." Although not opposed to all confirmatory trials, these criteria suggested to him "that trials designed mainly to demonstrate to others the benefits of a new therapy already thought to be effective may indeed be unethical."

The constitution of the Federal Republic of Germany includes legal recognition of the interests of the patient. The patient's right to self-determination enforces the obligation of the physician to make that person aware of the nature, importance, and implications of any planned procedure. The patient must be advised of "alternative methods of treatment if they differ in the degree of risk involved, in the range and gravity of their side effects, and in their prospects of success" (Eberbach, 1987). Also, the physician must include information about the assignment to a particular treatment being random.

> It is no solution to give information only after randomisation and only to those patients who will be undergoing the new therapy. It is true that patients in the control group receive the standard therapy but, in my opinion, it is wrong to infer that the ignorance of these patients concerning the additional randomisation is of no importance. [Eberbach, 1987]

Although the advancement of science may be weakened by legal requirements and professional ethical standards, this may be inescapable. Eberbach concludes, ". . . informing the patient is not simply necessary out of respect for (or even fear of) the courts. It is above all respect for the independent personality of the patient which makes this imperative."

Conclusions

Our position is that each comparative clinical trial should be designed with randomized or nonrandomized controls depending on the specific circumstances. As pointed out by Hill on several occasions, every method of control used for clinical trials has its defects. "No one method is best in every case, and the choice of method rests on consideration of the options and their consequences" (Cranberg, 1979).

The likelihood of an inadequate number of patients, lack or weakness of ethical justification, budget or time constraints, and the prospect of difficulty in obtaining informed consent for randomization may prohibit a randomized study. In an established sequence of cancer trials, some investigators may clearly prefer the advantages of a historical control plan and are willing to forgo the statistical superiority of a randomized design.

In 1976, Cornfield asked, "Does randomization provide the only basis by which a valid comparison can be achieved or is it simply an *ad hoc* device to achieve comparability between treatment groups?" So far, there has been no definitive answer as statisticians and clinicians continue to present their views on both sides.

Customarily, studies use randomized or nonrandomized controls, but not both. Pocock (1976) described a method for including historical controls into both the design and analysis of a randomized trial. He wrote that a valid historical control group should meet the following conditions:

1. Patients should have received a precisely defined standard treatment that was the same as that for the randomized controls.
2. Patients must have been part of a recent clinical study that had the same requirements for patient eligibility.
3. Methods of treatment evaluation must be the same.
4. Distributions of important patient characteristics in the group should be comparable with those in the new trial.
5. A previous study must have been performed in the same organization with largely the same clinical investigators.
6. There must be no other indications leading one to expect differing results between the randomized and historical controls.

These are stringent requirements, but some trials in sequence at cooperative cancer centers would probably qualify. In today's climate, the process of randomization may come under increasing attack.

> The challenge is to learn what we can from the scientific architecture of randomized trials and to use that knowledge to improve the structure of nonrandomized research. The splendid scientific contributions of randomized trials have made them the "gold standard" of cause/effect research—but when gold is too expensive or too difficult to obtain, we need to have good substitutes. [Feinstein, 1984]

All clinical trials, whether randomized or not, should be interpreted in a historical context. Both types of studies must be viewed in the light of previous and concurrent studies in the same area of research. Studies yielding results that are quite inconsistent with previous data will tend not to be accepted. The only real question is the extent to which formal account should be taken of previous studies in analyzing current data.

No clinical trial—whether randomized or not—is an entity unto itself. Each trial should be considered as part of an evolving research program. Confirmatory studies are essential for all clinical trials. If beneficial results are observed in a particular trial, they will not gain acceptance unless they can be repeated by other investigators who treat the same types of patients in a similar manner. This is especially relevant for historical control studies. Our belief is consistent with that of Dr. Emil Frei, III, coauthor of the first randomized clinical trial in cancer, who wrote

> I believe that each therapeutic hypothesis must be examined separately with respect to the experimental design, and a lot of damage has been done by pre-judging. People who insist that all studies must be randomized on the one hand, and those who insist that all studies should be historical control on the other, share one thing in common—they're both equally wrong. [Gehan, 1984, letter from Frei]

CHAPTER 6

Designs and Analyses of Studies of Historical Importance

Over the past 40 years, there has been an abundance of publications concerning methodology for the design and analysis of epidemiological investigations and clinical trials, and many examples of such research have been reported in the medical literature. In this chapter, we review some of the basic designs appropriate for epidemiological investigations and clinical trials and give examples of applications of the methodology. Because we work in cancer research, a field in which many of the contemporary designs were developed and applied, our examples are taken primarily from publications in oncology. We will be concerned with basic designs and analysis techniques that have proven useful and not with new ideas that, as far as we know, have not been tried.

Epidemiological Investigations: The Case–Control Study

A case–control study compares a group of people who have a specific disease (the cases) and a group of people with similar characteristics who do not have the disease (the controls) but who have been exposed to the possible risk factors for the disease in order to evaluate the hypothesis that one or more of the risk factors causes the disease. This study design is perhaps the dominant form used in analytical research in epidemiology, but it is not simplistic and cannot be done well without proper planning.

A Further Report on Cancer of the Breast, with Special Reference to Its Associated Antecedent Conditions (Janet Elizabeth Lane-Claypon, 1926)

The first case-control study of cancer may be Lane-Claypon's 1926 report, which Cole (1980) described as remarkably similar to a modern investigation. Lane-Claypon did not explain how she arrived at the case–control approach, but her study stood in a class by itself until after 1950 when her design was used for research in cancer epidemiology. Mantel and Haenszel (1959) judged her report significant because she set forth procedures for selecting matched hospital controls and related them to a consideration of study objectives. While case–control studies usually include one case and one control group, the design has been expanded to include two or more diseases (whose risk factors are believed to be similar) and two control groups (Cole, 1980).

Jerome Cornfield (1951) used Lane-Claypon's publication to illustrate a common stumbling block in medical research—the inability to achieve a truly representative control group. Lane-Claypon completed a long questionnaire on 508 postmenopausal women with breast cancer and on 509 similar control women who were hospitalized for noncancer illnesses and recorded the number of children born to women of each group. Her findings supported the association of increasing numbers of children with a lowered prevalence of breast cancer. Cornfield, however, wrote that Greenwood (in a previous analysis of Lane-Claypon's data) had "pointed out, without attaching any significance to it, that the control group had borne an average of about 25% more children than had all women in England and Wales with the same duration of marriage." Thus, it would appear that Lane-Claypon's control group was not representative of the general population. Hence, although hospital patients are often used as control subjects, they may not accurately reflect the frequency of a characteristic in the general population.

Smoking and Carcinoma of the Lung (Richard Doll and Austin Bradford Hill, 1950)

Doll and Hill's hallmark publication is included here because their design became the prototype for later case–control plans. As far as we know, their study was the first one concerning cancer that used two control groups. The study was organized because records in England and Wales showed a 15-fold increase in deaths from lung cancer between 1922 and 1947. Patients from 20 hospitals in the London area

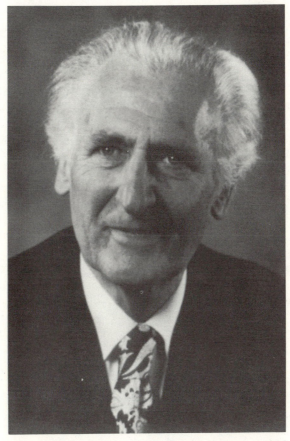

Sir Richard Doll. (From *Cancer Risks and Prevention*, M. P. Vessey and M. Gray (eds.), frontispiece. Copyright © 1985, Oxford University Press. Courtesy of Oxford University Press and Sir Richard Doll.)

participated, and an interviewer interrogated each patient having cancer of the lung, stomach, or large bowel. Those having cancer of the stomach or bowel served as the first control group. A second control group included hospital patients who did not have cancer but were the same sex and age as the patients with lung cancer and who were hospitalized at approximately the same time. Interviewers surveyed 649 men and 60 women with lung cancer and 649 men and 60 women with diseases other than cancer (Table 6.1). Of those with lung cancer, 0.3% of the men and 31.7% of the women were nonsmokers. The corresponding figures for the noncancer control group were men 4.2% and women 53.3%. The small percentage of nonsmoking men with lung cancer (0.3%) was certainly significantly less than the percentage (4.2%) in the noncancer control group. As will be shown in the next section, such data can be used to estimate the relative risk of lung cancer for smokers versus nonsmokers.

Adenocarcinoma of the Vagina: Association of Maternal Stilbestrol Therapy with Tumor Appearance in Young Women (Arthur L. Herbst, Howard Ulfelder, and David C. Poskanzer, 1971)

Although Herbst *et al.* introduced no innovative statistical technique in their study, we include it as an eloquent example of how powerful a very small, tight study can be; only eight patients were involved. A case–

Table 6.1. Numbers of Smokers and
Nonsmokers in Patients with Lung
Carcinoma and in Controls with Diseases
Other Than Cancer[a]

	Lung cancer	Controls
Males		
Smokers	647 (99.7%)	622 (95.8%)
Nonsmokers	2 (0.3%)	27 (4.2%)
Totals	649 (100%)	649 (100%)
Females		
Smokers	41 (68.3%)	28 (46.7%)
Nonsmokers	19 (31.7%)	32 (53.3%)
Totals	60 (100%)	60 (100%)

[a]Data from Doll, R., and Hill, A. B., 1950, Smoking and carcinoma of the lung. *Br Med J* 2:739–48, with permission.

control design was ideal in this instance because, although the exposure was rare, it was related to a high population-attributable risk percent (Cole, 1980). This assessment describes the "percentage of the group's total risk which is in excess of the risk among persons not exposed to the suspect factor" (Cole and MacMahon, 1971). "With diseases of low incidence, the controlled retrospective study may be the only feasible approach" (Mantel and Haenszel, 1959).

Adenocarcinoma of the vagina in young women had been recorded rarely before it was diagnosed in eight patients treated at two Boston hospitals between 1966 and 1969. The patients had not uniformly used any product that might have caused chronic irritation of the vagina. They had not used birth-control pills, and only one had sexual exposure. The cluster of cases prompted Herbst *et al.* to conduct a case–control investigation to determine the factors that might be associated with the genesis of the tumors.

Four matched controls for each patient were selected from the birth records of the hospital in which each patient was born. Females born within 5 days and on the same service as the patients with carcinoma were identified, and those born closest in time to the birth of each patient were selected. All mothers were interviewed.

Seven of the eight mothers of patients with carcinoma had received diethylstilbestrol, starting during the first trimester. No control mother had been given the synthetic estrogen ($p < 0.00001$). Herbst *et al.* found that maternal ingestion of diethylstilbestrol during early pregnancy apparently increased the risk of vaginal adenocarcinoma developing years later in the exposed daughter.

Estimation of Relative Risk

A Method of Estimating Comparative Rates from Clinical Data. Applications to Cancer of the Lung, Breast, and Cervix (Jerome Cornfield, 1951)

During the 1950s, statistical methods for the design and analysis of case–control studies were delineated. Cornfield explained that when one is trying to determine the association between possessing a certain characteristic and subsequently contracting a disease, one could choose comparable groups of persons having and not having the characteristic and calculate the percentage in each group who have or who develop the disease. This provides a true, or absolute, rate. For example, one could determine the percentage of cigarette smokers and nonsmokers who have or develop lung cancer. If a very sizable percentage of smokers develop lung cancer, tobacco would be regarded as a possible strong carcinogen.

This research plan is rarely used, however, because it is expensive and time consuming. Generally, like Doll and Hill (1950), one uses a group of people who have lung cancer and a second comparable group who do not and then one determines the percentage of cigarette smokers in each group. Instead of a true rate, this provides a relative frequency. Differences in relative frequencies do not give information about the strength of the association. Even if there were more smokers in the lung cancer group than in the noncancer group, that finding, by itself, would not suggest whether tobacco was a weak or a strong carcinogen.

In the Doll and Hill study of smoking and carcinoma of the lung, a major objective was to test the hypothesis that exposure to the risk factor of smoking increased the risk of developing lung cancer. However, the retrospective study of cases and controls allowed the calculation only of the relative frequency of being a smoker separately for cases and controls. One of the most important developments in the analysis of retrospective data was provided by Cornfield (1951) who demonstrated that the odds ratio(i.e., the ratio of the odds of being a smoker in the lung cancer cases to the odds of being a smoker in the control group) is an estimate of the approximate relative risk. Hence, inference procedures for the odds ratio and the approximate relative risk are the same for a retrospective study if the disease rate is low.

From the Doll and Hill study (Table 6.1), the odds of being a smoker were 99.7%/0.3% among the male patients with lung cancer and 95.8%/4.2% in the controls. Cornfield demonstrated that the ratio of these odds is an estimate of the approximate relative risk. Thus, one can infer from the Doll and Hill data that an estimate of the relative risk of lung cancer for smokers versus nonsmokers is 14.6 for men and 2.5 for women. Both of these risks are significantly higher than 1, which is the ratio that would be expected if smoking were not a risk factor.

The Mantel–Haenszel Procedure

Statistical Aspects of the Analysis of Data from Retrospective Studies of Disease (Nathan Mantel and William Haenszel, 1959)

A major concern for a statistician who is studying the extent of an association between a risk factor and the occurrence of a subsequent

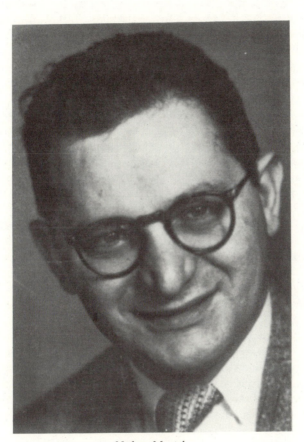

Nathan Mantel.

disease is the possibility of misleading associations. Cornfield's 1951 publication dealt with cases and controls that were essentially the same in all characteristics except the one being explored. Later, he and his colleagues wrote about controlling other variables (Wynder *et al.*, 1954).

Mantel and Haenszel considered controlling for the possibility of misleading associations, such as those posed by the presence of nuisance or confounding factors. One of the most important methods for control of confounding has been to divide the sample into a series of strata that are internally homogeneous with respect to the confounding factors. Separate relative risks calculated within each stratum are free of the bias arising from confounding. For example, we have seen that an estimate of relative risk can be obtained from Table 6.1 for both sexes. Mantel and Haenszel considered the problem of determining an overall estimate of relative risk from a series of 2×2 tables. Their procedure provides a summary relative risk over all tables in which the individual relative risks from each table are weighted according to their importance. A matched sample technique is one in which the number of stratifications equals the number of pairs of individuals. The classic paper by Mantel and Haenszel (1959) has provided the basis for the analysis of data from case–control studies; however, the proper application of the procedure requires that the population odds ratios do not vary greatly among the 2×2 tables.

If it is assumed that the relative risk of lung cancer among smokers is the same for males and females, then an overall estimate of relative risk for the Doll and Hill (1950) study is 4.52, which is between the estimate of 14.6 for males and 2.5 for females.

As noted in their title, Mantel and Haenszel wrote only about analyzing data from retrospective studies and stated, "A primary goal is to reach the same conclusions in a retrospective study as would have been obtained from a forward study, if one had been done." The Mantel–Haenszel statistic has been used extensively in epidemiologic and prospective studies and has also been applied to survival data (Mantel, 1966).

Epidemiological Investigations: Cohort Studies

Tumours of the Urinary Bladder in Workmen Engaged in the Manufacture and Use of Certain Dyestuff Intermediates in the British Chemical Industry. Part I. The Role of Aniline, Benzidine, Alpha-naphthylamine and Beta-naphthylamine

(R.A.M. Case, Marjorie E. Hosker, Drever B. McDonald,and Joan T. Pearson, 1954) and Part 2. *Further Consideration of the Role of Aniline and of the Manufacture of Auramine and Magenta (Fuchsine) as Possible Causative Agents* (R.A.M. Case and Joan T. Pearson, 1954).

Longitudinal studies in epidemiology are often labeled cohort studies. In a prospective project, one selects people who may be at risk of disease by some previous exposure or contact. Related information is collected, and the group is followed, sometimes for many years, while the occurrence of cancer and other diseases is duly recorded. In a historical study, one selects a group with a certain exposure experience and, by means of records and other information sources, determines how many of the subjects have gone on to develop cancer or other illnesses.

The 1954 articles by Case *et al.* and Case and Pearson from the Chester Beatty Institute became prototypes for historical cohort undertakings; these researchers were certainly creative and painstaking in their approach. Since the 1800s, it had been suspected that men working in the manufacture of aniline dyes might be at unusual risk of developing bladder cancer. A German surgeon, Ludwig Rehn, had reported that fuchsine workers were apt to develop tumors of the bladder. He believed that aniline was the culprit (Rehn, 1895). The term "aniline tumor of the bladder" was often used in the medical literature (Case *et al.*, 1954).

Case and his colleagues compiled a list of all workers employed for at least 6 months in the chemical industry in the United Kingdom between 1921 and 1952. Their study included 4622 men of different ages who were hired at different times by the 21 cooperating chemical companies. It was not possible to estimate the number of cases of bladder tumor that would be expected from the 4622 men if they incurred no special risk, but it was possible to estimate the number of death certificates mentioning tumor of the bladder that would be expected if no special risk occurred. The expected number was between three and five for the 4622 men, with allowances being made for their ages and dates of entry into the employing chemical companies. In 1952, the actual number of death certificates mentioning tumor of the bladder was 127. Thus, Case and colleagues' study provided data indicating that the workers' risk of dying of bladder tumor was approximately 30 times that of the general population.

In addition, Case (1953) described a method whereby one can get an idea of whether or not an environmental risk of bladder tumor exists in any occupation, assuming that the work records show the employee's name, age or date of birth, and hiring date. One must also know how many deaths from bladder tumor have in fact occurred. For the United Kingdom, Case published the tables required to complete these calculations. The Chester Beatty Institute still maintains a register of all males dying in England and Wales whose death certificates mention bladder tumor.

The Mortality of Doctors in Relation to their Smoking Habits. A Preliminary Report (Richard Doll and Austin Bradford Hill, 1954)

As far as we know, Doll and Hill's 1954 study was the first large prospective cohort study concerning cancer. In 1951, Doll and Hill noted that an association between smoking and lung cancer had been documented in many retrospective accounts, but the true nature of the connection remained unclear. They believed that an entirely new approach might provide further knowledge or detect some flaw in the previous research. They decided to launch a large prospective project to determine the frequency of the appearance of lung cancer among groups of people whose smoking habits were already known. They mailed a questionnaire to British physicians, and by the end of 1951, had received more than 40,000 replies from both male and female physicians.

Breslow and Day (1987) compared this endeavor with the researchers' previous (1950 and 1952) case–control plan, which took about 4½ years and included an analysis of 1465 patients with lung cancer and the same number of matched controls. The prospective study began in late 1951, and the results for men, based on 20 years or more of follow-up, were published in 1976 and 1978 (Doll and Peto), and those for women, based on 22 years of follow-up, in 1980 (Doll *et al.*). During those years, 441 and 27 deaths from lung cancer were recorded among the 34,440 men and 6194 women, respectively, enrolled in the study. Clearly, many more cases of cancer could be recorded in a shorter time in the case–control scheme with less than one-tenth of the persons questioned. However, this prospective study provided information on all causes of death and showed that there is nearly a twofold difference in the annual death rate between heavy smokers and nonsmokers. In addition, the study more clearly defined the effects of changing smoking habits and the time sequence of events (Breslow and Day, 1987).

In 1992, Doll wrote that when he and Richard Peto had published their 20 years' observations of male British physicians in 1976, they were able to determine the vital state of 99.7% of those who had replied to the initial inquiry. By the end of 1986, the cohort had been followed for 35 years, and significant trends in mortality with increasing numbers of cigarettes smoked were observed for 25 of the 48 causes of death examined. All of these causes were associated with smoking in British physicians (Doll, 1992).

Cohort studies have played a major role in the last 30 years in identifying specific environmental agents or other factors as carcinogenic hazards. Breslow and Day (1987) list about 40 agents or factors that have been identified, mainly through the conduct of cohort studies, as being causally related to cancer risk in man. Although the relative simplicity, low cost, and short time period over which they can be conducted make retrospective case–control studies the design of choice, there are clearly circumstances that require a design directed toward the continuous recording of events in the years prior to disease onset.

A major strength of the cohort study is that it gives a more complete picture of the health hazard associated with a given exposure to a risk factor. For example, lung cancer was established as being causally related to cigarette smoking, but identification of the spectrum of diseases for which smoking increases the risk came from a prospective study. Recall and selection bias can also usually be eliminated in a cohort study. For example, a retrospective study of children with cancer based on interviewing mothers of cases and controls regarding their pregnancies may clearly be subject to recall bias that would not be present in a cohort study.

Other strengths of cohort studies are (1) the effects of risk factors are more efficiently studied for exposures that are both rare in the general population and responsible for only a small proportion of a specific disease, (2) predisease data on biological parameters are available for study as potential risk factors, and (3) information obtained retrospectively may be too inaccurate to be of use.

The major limitations of cohort studies are that they require commitments of time, effort, and resources over a period of many years. Both individuals and funding agencies may be hesitant to embark on a project that will not yield results for a decade or more.

A recent development in cohort studies is a sampling of individuals within a cohort for comparison with controls (Prentice *et al.*, 1986). An example they cited is the analysis plan for the Women's Health Trial, which was undertaken in 1984 but discontinued in January 1988. The proposed project had been designed to include 32,000 participants (Greenwald, 1988; Prentice, 1991) randomly allocated to either their usual diet or a diet in which fat constituted only 20% of calories. Individuals were to be monitored by 4-day diet records and serum levels of micronutrients and hormones. Dietary data coding and biochemical analyses of blood sera on the entire cohort could have cost millions of dollars. Hence, it was proposed to analyze a subcohort of perhaps 20 or 25% of the entire cohort along with the approximately 5% of the cohort expected to develop breast cancer during follow-up. Thus, dietary records and blood sera would need to be collected for the entire cohort, but processed only for the subcohort and cases of breast cancer as they arose. Large cohort trials in disease prevention will probably use similar techniques in the future.

Clinical Trials

Randomized Trials

The historical background of the randomization technique was described in Chapter 3, highlighting the contributions of Fisher and Hill. Since their early innovations, the randomized clinical trial has been at the heart of medical clinical research. "The importance of randomized trials is their ability to convince the medical community . . . [without them] it is impossible truly to convince the scientific community about the efficacy of treatment" (Green, 1982). Also, "ethical considerations suggest that randomized trials are more suitable than uncontrolled experimentation in protecting the interests of patients. Randomized clinical trials remain the most reliable method for evaluating the efficacy of therapies" (Byar et al., 1976). In addition to the random allocation of treatment, blinding of both the patient and the investigator (double blinding) helps to minimize bias in a clinical trial.

A Comparative Study of Two Regimens of Combination Chemotherapy in Acute Leukemia (Emil Frei III, James F. Holland, Marvin A. Schneiderman, Donald Pinkel, George Selkirk, Emil J. Freireich, Richard T. Silver, G. Lennard Gold, and William Regelson, 1958)

The cooperative undertaking of Frei et al. is included here because it was the first prospective randomized clinical trial concerning cancer (acute leukemia) therapy in the United States; it followed the method

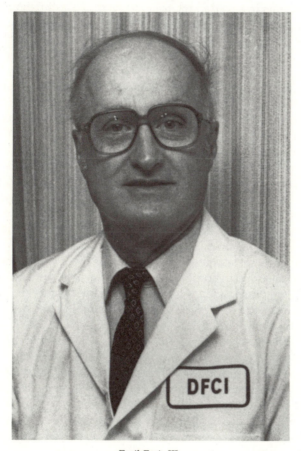

Emil Frei, III.

introduced by Bradford Hill. Researchers at the National Cancer Institute planned the trial in 1954 in cooperation with James Holland's group at Roswell Park Memorial Institute, Buffalo, New York. This was the first clinical trial reported by Leukemia Group B (subsequently Cancer and Leukemia Group B) sponsored by the National Cancer Institute.

All patients involved in the trial received two antimetabolite drugs (6-mercaptopurine and methotrexate) concurrently. For all patients, the dose of 6-mercaptopurine was started at 3.0 mg/kg daily. In the continuous group, 2.5 mg of methotrexate was given daily, and in the intermittent group, 7.5 mg of methotrexate was given every third day. The only difference between the two schedules was the timing of methotrexate; the total dosage of methotrexate was the same for each group. Criteria for the toxic effects expected to result from the drugs were clearly delineated in the protocol. If no toxic effects were apparent after 35 days, the dosage of both drugs was doubled.

Participants were subclassified by age (below or above 15 years), by type of leukemia (acute lymphocytic or myelocytic), and by history of antimetabolite therapy (yes or no). Within each of these categories patients were assigned by random allocation to either the continuous or intermittent schedule. The study was designed to provide about equal numbers of patients on each methotrexate dose regimen.

A nonparametric statistical test demonstrated that the median survival time and duration of remission were very similar for the two treatment regimens. Hence, the first reported cancer clinical trial reached an essentially negative conclusion about differences in outcome between the therapies.

The first randomized controlled trial of chemotherapy for solid malignant tumors compared nitrogen mustard and triethylene thiophosphoramide (Eastern Cooperative Group, 1960), and it, also, did not detect any difference in therapeutic efficacy between treatments.

Both of these early trials adopted certain principles that were subsequently followed in the cooperative group clinical trials program. These principles were cooperation of investigators from multiple centers in the planning and conduct of the trials, randomization of patients to therapies, careful evaluation of the outcomes of the patients, and statistical analysis of the results.

Sequential Designs

Experimentation may be broadly defined as sequential if its conduct at any stage depends on the results so far accumulated. In sequential medical trials, a decision is made to stop or continue at a particular monitoring time so that results influence the number of observations made. Conducting a sequential medical trial satisfies the ethical requirement that the trial should be stopped as soon as an important difference between treatments can be reliably demonstrated. Alternatively, a sequential design is sometimes chosen so that the trial can be stopped when continuance is very unlikely to demonstrate any important difference in therapeutic outcomes between therapies.

Generally, fewer observations are required for sequential designs than for fixed sample size designs. Whitehead (1983) stated that the time period from random allocation of therapy to an endpoint must be brief in relation to the interval for patient admission, or the benefit of early stopping will be forfeited. Also, the shorter length of sequential trials diminishes the amount of collateral data (e.g., long-term toxicity) that may be collected, so that such trials are most relevant when a single major endpoint can be chosen.

The identity of the person who first thought of sequential sampling is apparently not known. Dodge and Romig (1929) published a method of sampling inspection in which a second sample was to be drawn depending on the observations in the first sample (Wald, 1947). They originated this double-sampling plan to determine "whether a large lot of manufactured items is of good or poor quality as measured by the proportion of defectives" in the first sample. If the evidence were equivocal, a second sample would be inspected and a decision made based on the combined number of defective items. This is more efficient than the traditional single-sample procedure in reducing the number of items to be inspected (Ghosh, 1988). Walter Bartky (1943) extended the scheme to include more than two steps and Harold Hotelling (1941) mentioned chain or large-scale experiments designed to include successive stages. Abraham Wald (1947) regarded this latter idea as preliminary to sequential analysis.

Wald was a professor of mathematical statistics at Columbia University during World War II, and some of his work was directed by the National Defense Research Committee. According to Wald (1947), "The problem of sequential analysis arose in the Statistical Research Group at Columbia University in connection with some comments made by Captain G. L. Schuyler of the Bureau of Ordnance, Navy Department." Milton Friedman and W. Allen Wallis recognized the potentialities that sequential analysis might have for theoretical statistics, and they "exhibited a few examples of sequential modification of current test procedures resulting, in some cases, in an increase of efficiency" (Wald, 1947).

They proposed the problem of sequential analysis to Wald in March, 1943 (Weiss, 1988). In September of that year, Wald submitted a restricted and classified report, which subsequently led to his pioneering 1947 textbook, *Sequential Analysis*. In the book, he presented basic theory and worked out the sequential probability ratio test wherein items are inspected one by one and a decision is made at every step either to stop or continue the experiment. After the war, sequential analysis became useful in industrial procedures and was later adopted by medical statisticians.

Wald and his wife were killed in an airplane crash in India in 1950 when he was 48 years old (Reid, 1982, p. 228).

Irwin Bross (1952, 1953, 1958), of the Cornell University Medical College, wrote on the pros and cons of sequential procedures. In the 1952 article, he pointed out that in a clinical trial a sequential plan may be favored over a fixed sample size because (1) participants are paired and each outcome is analyzed as soon as it is reported; (2) less data may be required to reach a valid conclusion; and (3) much computing may be eliminated for research workers, many of whom do not have the services of full-time statisticians.

A sequential design incorporates rules for stopping or continuing the trial as results accumulate, so that the trial ends as soon as the recorded information is adequate to make a decision, saving time and effort as well as dollars and cents. "Rather more important is the ethical consideration, which requires that any unnecessary use of inferior treatments should be avoided" (Armitage, 1975). Although sequential designs may have some obvious advantages,

> Formal sequential methods have been applied in only a small fraction of actual [randomized clinical] trials. . . . few trials conform to the usual sequential design with two treatments, patient entry in matched pairs, instantaneous patient evaluation, a normal or binary response, and continuous surveillance of accumulating data. [Pocock, 1977]

In his book, *Sequential Medical Trials* (1960, 2nd ed., 1975), Peter Armitage outlined the basic principles of the sequential analysis technique and illustrated them with examples from medical trials.

The Effect of 6-Mercaptopurine on the Duration of Steroid-Induced Remissions in Acute Leukemia: A Model for Evaluation of Other Potentially Useful Therapy (Emil J. Freireich, Edmund Gehan, Emil Frei III, Leslie R.

Schroeder, Irving J. Wolman, Rachad Anbari, E. Omar Burgert, Stephen
D. Mills, Donald Pinkel, Oleg S. Selawry, John H. Moon, B. R. Gendel,
Charles L. Spurr, Robert Storrs, Farid Haurani, Barth Hoogstraten, and
Stanley Lee, 1963)

Freireich *et al.* conducted the first trial designed to test the worth of
a drug in prolonging remission in patients with acute leukemia. The
study design used a continuous variable (duration of remission) as
opposed to previous studies of remission induction that used a yes or
no variable. The study population consisted of 92 patients younger than
20 years; 62 had complete or partial remissions induced by cor-
ticosteroids. The patients at each of the 11 participating institutions were
paired according to remission status (complete or partial), and, by
random allocation, one member of the pair received 6-mercaptopurine
and the other received a placebo (given double-blind).

Patients now entered the remission maintenance phase of the
study, which was designed by Gehan, using a restricted (closed)
sequential scheme originated by Armitage (1957). This method was
chosen so that the trial could be stopped as soon as it was established
that one treatment was more effective in prolonging remission. The term
closed denotes that there was a fixed upper limit to the number of
participating patients. Nearly all medical trials are of the closed type,
whereas the original Wald sequential design had no such upper limit.

The study was planned to discriminate a proportion of preferences
of 0.75 favoring either therapy. If the true proportion of preferences for
6-mercaptopurine or placebo were 0.75, the probability of determining
that the correct therapy was in fact better was 0.95. If the null hypothesis
were true, there was a 0.95 probability that the outcome would reflect no
real difference. Figure 6.1 is a diagram of the working design.

When the first member of a pair relapsed from remission, a
preference was plotted for the treatment assigned to the partner, one
unit to the right and one up for a 6-mercaptopurine preference or one
unit to the right and one down for a placebo preference. If the path of
the plotted points crossed an upper (or lower) boundary, the outcome
favored 6-mercaptopurine (or placebo). If the path crossed the boundary
to the right, no real difference between treatments was indicated.

The study was stopped after the remission times of 21 pairs of
patients (42 patients) had been analyzed. Note that the path crossed the
upper boundary after 18 preferences and the trial could have been
closed at that time. However, data on remission status were collected at

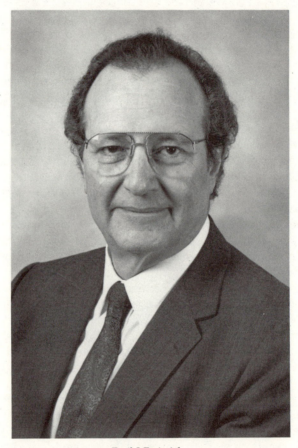

Emil J Freireich.

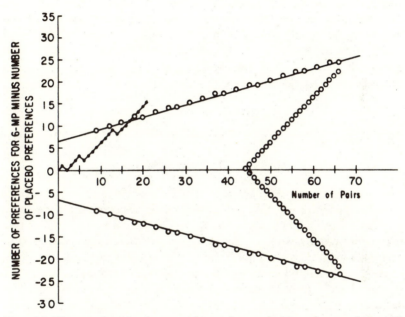

Figure 6.1. Diagram of restricted sequential procedure applied to preferences designed to be sensitive to proportion of 6-mercaptopurine or placebo preferences = 0.75. (From Freireich, E. J, Gehan, E. A., Frei, E. III, et al. 1963, with permission.)

3-month intervals, resulting in the delay. Survival of the two groups was not significantly different because patients receiving placebo were switched to 6-mercaptopurine when they relapsed. The capability of 6-mercaptopurine to prolong a corticosteroid-induced remission in patients with acute leukemia was clearly established in this sequential trial.

This study was influential because the researchers delineated a basic prototype that could be used for subsequent assessments of other agents. Further, the antileukemic activity of 6-mercaptopurine was detected without compromising the survival of the patients and for the first time, an agent's ability to maintain remission was studied separately from its remission-inducing activity. This study was the first prospective, randomized, double-blind, placebo-controlled sequential comparison of treatments in cancer research.

Analysis Techniques

Methods for Comparing Samples

Decision making in medical statistics is complex and one important aspect is deciding whether two or more samples come from the same population. A statistical significance test to compare outcomes of two treatment groups is an aid to medical decision making, but the hypothesis testing framework should not be viewed as a rigid rule for good science. As stated by Anscombe (1963), "The primary aim of the statistical analysis of the experiment should be to present as clearly and accurately as possible the evidence concerning relative effectiveness [of the treatments]." Significance levels have a prominent role in reporting the results of epidemiologic or clinical studies, but in almost all cases, confidence intervals for treatment differences are more informative than significance levels.

In 1908, W. S. Gosset (using the pseudonym "Student" because of the Guinness Company policy) developed a test of significance to determine whether a real difference exists between two average values obtained from paired data, without the assumption of known variability. In his example, 12 patients took part in an experiment, each of whom received two treatments to induce sleep, and Student's *t* test established that the additional hours of sleep gained by one of the treatments was significantly greater than the other. Fisher later extended this test to include the comparison of average values from two independent samples.

Karl Pearson (1900) was the originator of the chi-square statistic which may be used to test for an association between factors in retrospective case–control studies or to test the difference between proportions in retrospective or prospective studies. Chi-square tests are used when the data to be analyzed are qualitative, such as differences in response rate, and such tests have been developed for independent samples, matched samples, and two independent samples, adjusting for differences in a subclassification such as age.

Frank Wilcoxon, in the landmark publication *Individual Comparisons by Ranking Methods* (1945), was the originator of statistical techniques for dealing with ranked observations, and it was later established that replacing the numerical values of observations by their ranks in the sample was almost as efficient as using the observations themselves. There was a follow-up article in *Biometrics* (Wilcoxon, 1947) wherein he considered the two-sample form of the rank-sum statistic with samples of equal size. In their short biography of him, Bradley and Hollander (1988) report that Wilcoxon was born in Ireland in 1892 to wealthy American parents. He grew up in Catskill, New York, and after World War I, he earned a Master of Science degree in chemistry from Rutgers University and a doctoral degree in physical chemistry from Cornell University. For the next 25 years, Wilcoxon researched fungicides and insecticides at the Boyce Thompson Institute for Plant Research, the Nichols Copper Company, and the American Cyanamid Company.

After studying Fisher's first book in 1925, Wilcoxon developed a lively interest in statistics that eventually led to his many contributions to rank tests and multiple comparison procedures. His most influential article was that written in 1945 (already mentioned) in which he presented two rank tests: the rank-sum test for the two-sample problem and the signed-rank test for paired samples. This work was at the forefront of the subsequent evolution of nonparametric statistics. Kruskal and Wallis (1952) extended the rank-sum test to the problem of more than two samples.

In experiments, there may be

> more than just one or two conditions (treatments, etc.) under investigation. Often multiple hypotheses need to be tested. In such

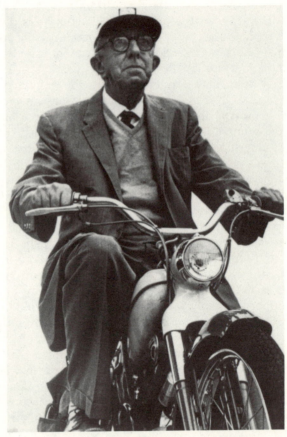

Frank Wilcoxon. (Courtesy of Dr. Fred Leysieffer, professor and chairman, Department of Statistics, Florida State University, Tallahassee.)

settings, it is important to control the overall or experimentwise error rate. Wilcoxon recognized this and had a strong interest in multiple comparisons. In particular, his 1964 revision of the booklet *Some Rapid Approximate Statistical Procedures* (joint with Roberta A. Wilcox) features multiple comparison procedures based on Wilcoxon rank sums. . . . The booklet played a significant role in the [later] widespread use of nonparametric multiple comparison procedures. [Bradley and Hollander, 1988]

Mann and Whitney of Ohio State University put forward an alternative version of the Wilcoxon test in 1947 that was based on comparing every observation in one sample with every observation in the other, scoring +1 if the observation were greater or −1 if the observation were less and basing a test statistic on the sum of all comparisons. It turns out that this test is equivalent to the Wilcoxon test, and Gehan (1965) presented a variant of this test, a distribution-free two-sample test that extended the Wilcoxon test to survival data, in which there may be arbitrary or random censoring on the right. In the context of survival data, there is censoring on the right when the observation of the person in the trial is ended before the person experiences the endpoint. This may happen if the individual is lost to follow-up before the endpoint occurs or if individuals enter the study over a period of time and analysis is carried out at some fixed time after the start of the study.

Life-Table Analysis

The calculus of probabilities may be the oldest of statistical methods. The underlying theories were established and the first introductory book was written in the mid-1600s. At about the same time, Petty and Graunt grasped the elementary principles of the life table, and by 1693, Halley had introduced mortality tables (see Chapter 1).

The proper principles for setting up life tables were worked out by actuaries in Britain in the first half of the 19th century. The tables were developed from population and insurance records (Lew, 1985), originally for insurance companies. Farr's contributions in the area of vital statistics and mortality tables during this period are summarized in Chapter 2.

Clinical trials often are conducted over a period of several years and have endpoints of the survival type, such as progression-free survival time, or time from start of study to experiencing some event (e.g., myocardial infarction or stroke). Hence, representation of the distribution of survivals for a group of patients is a common problem. The elementary statistical method of calculating a sample mean is not applicable because some patients will not have died at the time of analysis. Ordinarily, the data will contain some right-censored observations that are known only to be at least as great as the observed values for the patients still under observation.

The most common way of representing such data is to estimate the survival function $S(t)$. This function gives the probability of surviving more than t time units, where t is measured from the start of treatment, time of diagnosis, or date of randomization. There are basically two satisfactory methods for estimating $S(t)$: the life table or actuarial method often attributed to Berkson and Gage (1950) and the maximum likelihood (or product limit) method of Kaplan and Meier (1958).

Berkson and Gage were the first to publish simple explanations of procedures for estimating a survival function in the presence of right-censored data; their method is most applicable when the number of patients is large. Joseph Berkson was an epidemiologist, statistician, and physician at the Mayo Clinic who made important contributions to life-table analysis and minimum logit chi-square procedures. In the 1950 article, he and Gage outlined simple step-by-step procedures for calculating survival rates for cancer.

The Kaplan and Meier (1958) method also provides an estimate of the proportion, $S(t)$, of patients whose age at death would exceed t if no patients had been censored. This is a maximum likelihood estimate, also known as a product-limit estimate. An early version of the method was given by Böhmer in 1912 (Buckland, 1964).

Both life-table methods make the important assumption that the survival experience of censored patients subsequent to time of censoring is the same as that for patients who have remained under follow-up. This assumption should be examined in each application. A bias could arise, for example, if, for some reason, censored patients were more (or less) likely to die a short time after censoring than patients who remained under follow-up.

It is of interest that survival time can be described by three functions that are mathematically equivalent in the sense that, given any one of the functions, the other two can be derived, even though the three characterize different aspects of the data. Formulas have been given to demonstrate this (Broadbent, 1958; Cox, 1962; Buckland, 1964, pp. 11–35; and Gehan, 1969).

1.   The survivorship function $S(t)$ characterizes the proportion of individuals surviving more than t time units and can be used to obtain median or other percentile estimates of survival time. For example, one can estimate the proportion of patients with a disease surviving longer than 5 years. As has been explained, estimates of the survivorship function can be made using the life-table method of Berkson and Gage or the product-limit estimate of Kaplan and Meier.

2.   The hazard function, or age-specific failure rate, is the limit of the probability of nearly immediate failure for an individual known to be alive at time t. A plot of the hazard function describes the aging of the study population. When the risk of death per unit time remains constant with time, there is no aging and survival time will be exponentially distributed. Plotting the hazard function for a set of data aids in making a choice of theoretical survival distribution for modeling the data.

3.   The probability density function can be used to estimate the proportion of deaths that will occur during any time interval and/or to estimate highs or lows in the frequency of death.

Multivariate Regression Analysis

The relative evaluation of therapies in a clinical trial should take into account all patient characteristics that may influence outcome. In addition to the therapies under investigation, features associated with the natural history of the disease may also influence outcome. For example, in breast cancer trials, survival is influenced by menopausal status, nodal involvement, tumor size, and estrogen receptor status. By the techniques of multivariate analysis, it is possible to compare therapies, taking into account the prognostic factors of the patients. Statistical models are used to incorporate these covariates (patient characteristics) into the analysis. General statistical models have been developed for both categorical and survival data. The models ordinarily used for these two endpoints are referred to as logistic and proportional hazards models, respectively, though the latter model is often called the "Cox model" in honor of Sir David Roxbee Cox.

Cox wrote seminal papers concerning both logistic regression, *The Regression Analysis of Binary Sequences* (1958), and proportional hazards regression, *Regression Models and Life Tables* (1972), which won him the General Motors prize in cancer treatment research in 1990. His technique has been used in many clinical trials in which survival-type

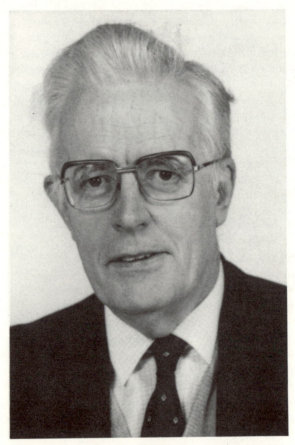

Sir David Roxbee Cox.

endpoints are compared between therapies, taking into account the major patient features related to outcome.

The basic ideas of these models will be presented, assuming that two therapies are being compared and adjusting for a single covariate; generalization to many covariates is described in the original papers.

Logistic Regression Models

Suppose there are two therapies (A and B) having true response probabilities p_α and p_β that are unknown. The odds of response for each therapy is defined as the ratio of the probability of response to the probability of no response, i.e., p_α/q_α and p_β/q_β where $q_\alpha = 1 - p_\alpha$ and $q_\beta = 1 - p_\beta$. Assume that a clinical trial were conducted comparing treatments A and B, where the primary endpoint was the complete response rate and it was desired to test the difference between two treatments adjusting for the ages of the patients. If X_1 denotes the treatment group ($X_1 = 0$ for treatment A and $X_1 = 1$ for treatment B) and X_2 denotes the age group ($X_2 = 0$ for younger ages and $X_2 = 1$ for older ages), then the logistic model assumes that the log of the odds ratio takes the following form:

$$\log(p/q) = \alpha_0 + \alpha_1 X_1 + \alpha_2 X_2$$

where α_0, α_1, and α_2 are unknown parameters in the model. In this formulation, $p_\alpha = e^{\alpha_0}/(1 + e^{\alpha_0})$, with corresponding terms for the other probabilities. The functional form of p_α is the logistic function, and hence, the term *logistic model*.

The logarithms of the odds ratios for the four types of patients are given in Table 6.2. Note that the model is additive on the log scale and that hypotheses about the influence of treatment and age group correspond to tests of significance concerning the parameters of the model.

The parameters α_0, α_1, and α_2 in the model are unknown, but may be estimated from the data. Also, it is possible to test the significance of each α value, although the most interesting is usually whether a particular α value is 0. Having estimates of the α values permits a logical interpretation of the data in the context of the model assumed. For example, if $\alpha_2 = 0$, then age is not a prognostic factor and the estimated response rates for older and younger patients on both treatments would be the same. If $\alpha_1 = 0$, then the response rates for both treatments would be the same. The estimate of α_1 provides a measure of the difference in response rates between the two treatments, taking into account the age

*Table 6.2. Logistic Regression Model
for the Four Groups of Patients*

Treatment	Age	Logistic model
A	Younger	$\log\left(\dfrac{p_\alpha}{q_\alpha}\right) = \alpha_0$
B	Younger	$\log\left(\dfrac{p_\beta}{q_\beta}\right) = \alpha_0 + \alpha_1$
A	Older	$\log\left(\dfrac{p_\alpha}{q_\alpha}\right) = \alpha_0 + \alpha_2$
B	Older	$\log\left(\dfrac{p_\beta}{q_\beta}\right) = \alpha_0 + \alpha_1 + \alpha_2$

distribution of the patients on the two therapies. In fitting the model to some actual data in a clinical trial, it is important to demonstrate that the model provides a good fit to the experimental data.

Prognostic Factors in Acute Leukemia (Edmund A. Gehan, Terry L. Smith, Emil J. Freireich, Gerald P. Bodey, Victorio Rodriguez, John Speer, and Kenneth B. McCredie, 1976)

Gehan *et al.* accomplished an extensive analysis of the patient characteristics related to the prognosis of this disease by studying 424 previously untreated adults with acute leukemia. Survival time was analyzed in addition to the probability of remission. They considered 17 covariates (e.g., age, type of leukemia, organomegaly) and used logistic regression analysis (Cox, 1970) to develop a statistical model relating the covariates to the complete remission rate. The regression coefficients were established in a stepwise manner so that the first patient characteristic was the most influential variable in predicting remission, the second characteristic the second most influential (assuming the first was in the equation), and so on.

For patients with no prior treatment, the most important characteristics related to probability of complete remission were age, temperature status at start of study, hemoglobin value, and platelet count. Favorable values of these covariates were young age, temperature < 100°F, hemoglobin > 12 g/100 ml, and platelet count > 100,000/mm^3. Since these early studies, extensive analyses have been conducted in leukemia research (Keating *et al.*, 1980; T. L. Smith *et al.*, 1982).

Proportional Hazards Regression

A primary endpoint in many clinical trials is the time until the occurrence of an event such as death or disease progression. The statistical analysis of such survival data requires the use of special methods because the event may not have occurred in all patients when the data are analyzed. In a classic publication, Cox (1972) extended the concepts of regression analysis to survival data. His proportional hazards regression model provides a methodology for assessing the simultaneous association between multiple patient characteristics and survival.

Suppose a clinical trial were conducted comparing two treatments, A and B, where the primary endpoint was survival time and it was desired to test the difference between the treatments adjusting for the ages of the patients. If X_1 denotes treatment group ($X_1 = 0$ for treatment A and $X_1 = 1$ for treatment B) and X_2 denotes age group ($X_2 = 0$ for younger ages and $X_2 = 1$ for older ages), then Cox's model assumes that the hazard function for a patient takes the form

$$h_0(t) \cdot e^{\beta_1 X_1 + \beta_2 X_2}$$

where $h_0(t)$ is a baseline hazard function, or a hazard function for a reference group, assuming $X_1 = X_2 = 0$. Here, β_1 and β_2 are unknown regression coefficients that can be estimated from the data. The hazard functions for the four types of patients are shown in Table 6.3.

Note that these hazard functions are multiples of one another differing only because of the multiplicative exponential term. If ratios of hazard functions are estimated, it is not necessary to know the baseline hazard $h_0(t)$ to compare the four groups. The hypothesis that treatment group is not associated with survival is given by testing whether $\beta_1 = 0$,

Table 6.3.   Cox Regression Model for the Four Groups of Patients

Treatment	Age	Hazard function
A	Younger	$h_0(t)$
B	Younger	$h_0(t)e^{\beta_1}$
A	Older	$h_0(t)e^{\beta_2}$
B	Older	$h_0(t)e^{\beta_1+\beta_2}$

whereas the hypothesis that age group is not associated with survival corresponds to $\beta_2 = 0$. The coefficients β_1 and β_2 can be estimated from the data without any assumptions concerning $h_0(t)$.

The analysis of survival data using Cox's model consists of estimating the parameters β_1 and β_2 with their standard errors. This permits the estimation of relative risks of survival in the various groups, the construction of confidence intervals for the parameters or relative risks, and tests of hypotheses about the β values. Generalizations of Cox's model have been made for multiple explanatory variables, use of stratification, the inclusion of explanatory variables that can vary with time (i.e., time-dependent covariates), and interaction terms. In applications, there should be verification of whether the proportional hazards assumption is correct and whether or not interaction terms are of importance. A comprehensive presentation of the theoretical aspects of the model is given by Cox and Oakes (1984).

Obesity: An Adverse Prognostic Factor for Patients Undergoing Adjuvant Chemotherapy for Breast Cancer (Jorge Bastarrachea, Gabriel N. Hortobagyi, Terry L. Smith, Shu-Wan C. Kau, and Aman U. Buzdar, 1994)

A retrospective review of the characteristics and clinical course of 735 patients with stage II or III primary breast carcinoma treated on postoperative adjuvant chemotherapy protocols was undertaken to determine whether obesity is an independent prognostic factor among women with node-positive breast cancer. Also, the relationship of obesity to other prognostic factors, such as menopausal status, stage of disease, and involvement of lymph nodes, was investigated. Endpoints were disease-free survival and overall survival, but since conclusions were similar, results will be given only for disease-free survival. The estimated 10-year disease-free rate for patients not more than 20% over ideal weight was 54% compared with 40% for remaining patients (classified as obese) ($p < 0.01$). Obesity was significantly associated with postmenopausal status, stage III tumors, and tumors > 5 cm in diameter. Hence, obese patients tended to be at a higher risk for disease recurrence because of other prognostic features. In this application the hazard function has the form

$$h_0(t) \cdot e^{\beta_1 X_1 + \beta_2 X_2 + \beta_3 X_3 + \beta_4 X_4}$$

where the covariates are coded as follows:

• Obesity ($X_1 = 0$ for nonobese, $X_1 = 1$ for obese)

- Menopausal status ($X_2 = 0$ for pre, $X_2 = 1$ for post)
- Stage ($X_3 = 0$ for II, $X_3 = 1$ for III)
- Nodes involved ($X_4 = 0$ for ≤ 3, $X_4 = 1$ for 4–10, $X_4 = 2$ for > 10)

A Cox regression analysis was performed to adjust for differences in disease characteristics between obese and nonobese patients, and the results are shown in Table 6.4.

After accounting for other prognostic features, the relative risk of disease recurrence among obese patients was 1.33 compared with the nonobese population. The increased risk associated with obesity was not as great as that for stage III disease or the presence of more than 10 involved nodes. In this application, extent of the interaction effect between obesity and other prognostic factors was examined by considering the addition of interaction terms between obesity and stage of disease, nodal status, and menopausal status. This analysis of interaction effect demonstrated the importance of obesity as a prognostic factor for patients with stage III disease. It also confirmed the importance of the stage of disease and the involvement of lymph nodes as prognostic factors and demonstrated that obesity is associated with a higher risk of disease recurrence, independently of the other factors.

Metanalysis

Review of the medical literature on a specific subject has frequently been included in the introductory section of research articles. It is also

Table 6.4. Elements of Proportional Hazard Model

Covariate	Level	Hazard function	Estimates of risk Ratio	p
Obese (% over ideal weight)	≤20%	$h_O(t)$	1	
	>20%	$h_O(t)e^{\beta_1}$	1.33 (1.05 to 1.68)[a]	0.02
Menopausal status	Pre	$h_O(t)$	1	
	Post	$h_O(t)e^{\beta_2}$	1.17 (0.95 to 1.45)	0.14
Stage	II	$h_O(t)$	1	
	III	$h_O(t)e^{\beta_3}$	1.51 (1.21 to 1.89)	<0.01
Nodes involved	≤3	$h_O(t)$	1	
	4–10	$h_O(t)e^{\beta_4}$		
	>10	$h_O(t)e^{2\beta_4}$	1.58 (1.38 to 1.82)	<0.01

[a]95% confidence interval for risk ratio.

common to have an entire paper, monograph, or book devoted to such a compendium or summary. The difference between metanalysis and an ordinary scientific review is that the latter tends to be personal, reflecting the views of the reviewer. On the other hand, metanalysis refers to the use of formal statistical techniques to sum up the quantitative evidence from separate studies designed to investigate the same hypothesis. The end product is a summary estimate of a quantity that reflects a difference in the effectiveness of treatments or methods.

Researchers are often unable to recruit enough patients into a randomized clinical trial to reveal a small but potentially meaningful difference. When the results of a collection of such studies are assembled, however, the total number of patients may be adequate to demonstrate a real difference in effectiveness between treatments.

> The potential usefulness of meta-analysis is highlighted when we learn that at least half of one series of "negative" therapeutic trials had a statistical power of 60% or less (type II error of 40% or more) because the study groups were too small [Cunningham, 1988]

Ellenberg (1988) attributes the introduction of the term *metanalysis* to Glass (1976). Metanalytic methods were first used in psychology and education, but statisticians in medical research soon took up the procedure. In 1992, Sacks *et al.* surveyed 164 metanalyses of randomized controlled trials and used a scoring method to evaluate their quality.

The principal difficulties in applying metanalysis to clinical trials relate to differences among therapies, study designs, patient populations, follow-up times, and quality of the studies. The studies will have been done at different times, and methods of analysis may differ. In using metanalysis, the statistician may resort to complex techniques (e.g., weighting schemes for combining results from different studies). The summary endpoint may involve various measures of treatment effect such as the difference in number of deaths between treatment and control groups or the ratio of treatment group to control group mortality rates. The advantage of metanalysis is that the summary measure of treatment effect should have smaller variability (because of the large number of patients and studies) than that of any individual study.

Richard Peto and colleagues have been proponents of metanalysis using the technique to summarize various aspects of medical studies. He and his associates believe that "in order to avoid selective biases and to minimize random errors, inference about the effects of treatment on

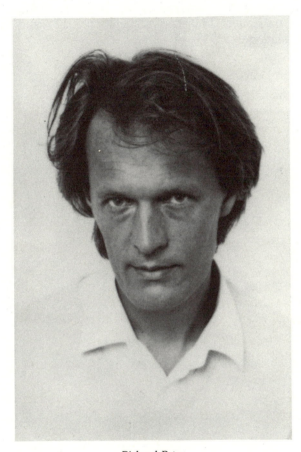

Richard Peto.

serious endpoints needs to be based not on one, or a few, of the available trial results, but on a systematic overview of the totality of the evidence from all the relevant unconfounded randomized trials" (Collins *et al.*, 1987). They have used the techniques of metanalysis to review breast cancer (Cuzick *et al.*, 1987, 1988), heart disease (MacMahon *et al.*, 1988, 1990; Yusuf *et al.*, 1988; Collins *et al.*, 1990; Chen *et al.*, 1991), antiplatelet treatment (Antiplatelet Trialists' Collaboration, 1988), and the use of heparin (Collins *et al.*, 1988).

References

Advisory Committee to the Surgeon General of the Public Health Service, 1964, *Smoking and Health*. Washington, D.C.: U. S. Government Printing Office, Publication No. 1103.

Amberson, J. B., Jr., McMahon, B. T., and Pinner, M., 1931, A clinical trial of sanocrysin in pulmonary tuberculosis. *Am Rev Tuberc* **24**:401–35.

Andersen, P. K., 1985, Time-dependent covariates and Markov processes. In *Modern Statistical Methods in Chronic Disease Epidemiology*, S. H. Moolgavkar, R. L. Prentice (eds.). New York: John Wiley & Sons, p. 82.

Anderson, M., 1989, Expanding the influence of the Statistical Association: American Statistical Association from 1880 to 1930. In *Proc Am Stat Assoc Sesquicentennial Invited Papers Session* pp. 561–75.

Anderson, R. L., Monroe, R. J., and Nelson, L. A., 1979, Gertrude M. Cox: A modern pioneer in statistics. *Biometrics* **35**:3–7.

Angell, M., 1984, Patients' preferences in randomized clinical trials. *N Engl J Med* **310**:1385–87.

Anscombe, F. J., 1963, Sequential medical trials. *J Am Stat Assoc* **58**:365–83.

Antiplatelet Trialists' Collaboration, 1988, Secondary prevention of vascular disease by prolonged antiplatelet treatment. *Br Med J* **296**:320–31.

Areen, J., and King, P., 1990, Legal regulation of human gene therapy. *Hum Gene Ther* **1**:151–61.

Armitage, P., 1957, Restricted sequential procedures. *Biometrika* **44**:9–26.

Armitage, P., 1960, *Sequential Medical Trials*. London: Blackwell, p. ix, 2nd ed. 1975.

Armitage, P., 1982, The role of randomization in clinical trials. *Stat Med* **1**:345–52.

Armitage, P., 1984, A toast to the Royal Society on the 150th anniversary of the Royal Statistical Society. *J R Stat Soc A* **147**(2):126.

Armitage, P., 1990, The editorship of *Biometrika*. *Biometrika* **77**:4.

Arrow, K. J., 1988, Comment. *Stat Sci* **3**:90–91.

Atkins, H., 1966, Conduct of a controlled clinical trial. *Br Med J* **2**:377–79.

Avicenna, 1486, *Canon*. Venice: Impensis Petri Maufer.

Bacon, F., 1627, *Sylva Sylvarum, or a Natural History*. London: William Rawley, pp. 109–10.

Bancroft, T. A., 1972, *Statistical Papers in Honor of George W. Snedecor*. Ames: Iowa State University Press, pp. ix–xvii.

Banta, H. D., 1982, RCTs and the federal government. *Controlled Clin Trials* 3:173–83.

Bartky, W., 1943, Multiple sampling with constant probability. *Ann Math Stat* 14:363–77.

Bartlett, E., 1848, *An Inquiry into the Degree of Certainty in Medicine and into the Nature and Extent of its Power over Disease*. Philadelphia: Lea & Blanchard, pp. 30–43.

Bastarrachea, J., Hortobagyi, G. N., Smith, T. L., *et al.*, 1994, Obesity: An adverse prognostic factor for patients undergoing adjuvant chemotherapy for breast cancer. *Ann Intern Med* 120:18–25.

Baxby, D., 1981, *Jenner's Smallpox Vaccine: The Riddle of Vaccinia Virus and its Origin*. London: Heinemann, pp. 1–9.

Bayes, T., 1731, *Divine Benevolence, or an Attempt to Prove That the Principal End of the Divine Providence and Government is the Happiness of His Creatures*. London.

Bayes, T., 1736, *An Introduction to the Doctrine of Fluxions, and a Defence of the Mathematicians Against the Objections of the Author of The Analyst*. London.

Bayes, T., 1763, An essay towards solving a problem in the doctrine of chances. *Philos Trans* 53:370–418. Reprinted in *Biometrika* 45:293–315, 1958.

Bellhouse, D., 1993, The role of roguery in the history of probability. *Stat Sci* 8:410–20.

Bennett, J. H., 1983, Darwin–Fisher correspondence 1915–1929. In *Natural Selection, Heredity, and Eugenics*, J. H. Bennett (ed.). London: Oxford University Press (Clarendon), pp. 116–17.

Berkman, S., 1991, Volunteering for medical research. *Good Housekeeping*, August, p. 165.

Berkson, J. B., and Gage, R. R., 1950, Calculation of survival rates for cancer. *Proc Staff Meet Mayo Clin* 25:270–86.

Bernoulli, D., 1738a, Specimen theoriae novae de mensura sortis. *Commentarii Academiae Imperialis Petropolitanae* 5:175–92 (for the years 1730–31).

Bernoulli, D., 1738b, *Hydrodynamica, sive de viribus et motibus fluidorum commentarii*. Strasbourg.

Bernoulli, D., 1766, Essai d'une nouvelle analyse de la mortalité causée par la petite vérole et les avantages de l'inoculation pour la prévenir. *Histoire de l'Acad. Royale des Sciences, Année 1760, avec des Mémoires de Mathématique et de Physique pour la même Année*, Paris.

Bernoulli, D., 1777, *The Most Probable Choice Between Several Discrepant Observations and the Formation Therefrom of the Most Likely Induction*. In Latin in the memoirs of the Academy of St. Petersburg, *Acta Acad Petrop* pp. 3–33. Translated by C. G. Allen and reprinted in *Biometrika* 48:3–13, 1961.

Berry, A., 1898, *A Short History of Astronomy*. London: John Murray, p. 240. Reprinted New York: Dover, 1961.

Böhmer, P. E., 1912, Theorie der unabhängigen Wahrscheinlichkeiten. *Rapports, Mémoires et Procès-verbaux de Septième. Congrès International d'Actuaires* (Amsterdam) 2:327–43.

Bonchek, L. I., 1979, Are randomized trials appropriate for evaluating new operations? *N Engl J Med* 301:44–45.

Bowler, R. G., Buckell, M., Garrad, J., and Hill, A. B., 1947, Risk of fluorosis in magnesium factories. *Br J Ind Med* 4:216–22.

Box, J. F., 1978, *R. A. Fisher: The Life of a Scientist*. New York: John Wiley & Sons, pp. 77–78.

Box, J. F., 1981, Gosset, Fisher, and the *t* distribution. *Am Stat* 35:61–66.

Box, J. F., 1983, Ronald Aylmer Fisher (1890–1962). In *Encyclopedia of Statistical Sciences*, vol. 3, S. Kotz, N.L.Johnson (eds.). New York: John Wiley & Sons, pp.103–11.

Bradley, R. A., 1988, Comment: Harold Hotelling's views on statistics. *Stat Sci* 3:98–103.

Bradley, R. A., and Hollander, M., 1988, Frank Wilcoxon. In *Encyclopedia of Statistical Sciences*, vol.9, S. Kotz, N. L. Johnson (eds.). New York: John Wiley & Sons, pp. 609–12.

Breslow, N. E., and Day, N. E., 1987, The role of cohort studies in cancer epidemiology. In *Statistical Methods in Cancer Research*, vol. II. Lyon: International Agency for Research on Cancer, pp. 2–46.

Broadbent, S., 1958, Simple mortality rates. *Appl Stat* 7:86–95.

Bross, I. D. J., 1952, Sequential medical plans. *Biometrics* 8:188–205.

Bross, I. D. J., 1953, *Design for Decision*. New York: Macmillan Co.

Bross, I. D. J., 1958, Sequential clinical trials. *J Chronic Dis* 8:349–65.

Brown, B. W., Jr., 1970, The use of controls in the clinical evaluation of cancer therapies. In *NCI Symposium on Statistical Aspects of Protocol Design*, pp. 161–79.

Buckland, W. R., 1964, *Statistical Assessment of the Life Characteristic: A Bibliographic Guide*, M. G. Kendall (ed.). New York: Hafner, p. 75.

Buffon, G.-L. L., 1777, *Essai d'Arithmétique Morale*.

Bull, J. P., 1959, The historical development of clinical therapeutic trials. *J. Chronic Dis* 10:218–48.

Byar, D. P., 1991, Comment on R. M. Royall: Ethics and statistics in randomized clinical trials. *Stat Sci* 6:65–68.

Byar, D. P., Simon, R. M., Friedewald, W. T., *et al.*, 1976, Randomized clinical trials: Perspectives on some recent ideas. *N Engl J Med* 295:74–80.

Cancer Chemotherapy National Service Center, 1960, The national program of cancer chemotherapy research. *Cancer Chemother Rep* 1:5–34.

Case, R. A. M., 1953, The expected frequency of bladder tumour in works populations. *Br J Ind Med* 10:114–20.

Case, R. A. M., and Pearson, J. T., 1954, Tumours of the urinary bladder in workmen engaged in the manufacture and use of certain dyestuff intermediates in the British chemical industry. Part II. Further consideration of the role of aniline and of the manufacture of auramine and magenta (fuchsine) as possible causative agents. *Br J Ind Med* 11:213–16.

Case, R. A. M., Hosker, M. E., McDonald, D. B., *et al.*, 1954, Tumours of the urinary bladder in workmen engaged in the manufacture and use of certain dyestuff intermediates in the British chemical industry. Part I. The role of aniline, benzidine, alpha-naphthylamine and beta-naphthylamine. *Br J Ind Med* 11:75–104.

Celsus, A. C., 1478, *De Medicina*, translated by W. J. Spencer. London: Heinemann, 1935. Reported in J. P. Bull, p. 220, 1959.

Chang, W.-C., 1976, Statistical theories and sampling practice. In *On the History of Statistics and Probability*, D. B. Owen (ed.). New York: Marcel Dekker, pp. 299–315.

Chen, Z., Peto, R., Collins, R., *et al.*, 1991, Serum cholesterol concentration and coronary heart disease in population with low cholesterol concentrations. *Br Med J* 303: 276–82.

Chow, V. T., 1966, Bernoulli's law. In *Encyclopedia International*, vol. 2. New York: Grolier, pp. 546–47.

Cobbett, W., 1800, *The Rush-light*. A monograph. New York: William Cobbett, February 28.

Cochran, W. G., 1934, The distribution of quadratic forms in a normal system. *Proc Cambridge Philos Soc* 30:178–91.

Cochran, W. G., 1938, Long-term agricultural experiments. *J R Stat Soc Suppl* 6:104–48.

Cochran, W. G., 1946, Relative accuracy of systematic and stratified random samples for a certain class of populations. *Ann Math Stat* **17**:164–77.

Cochran, W. G., 1947a, Some consequences when the assumptions for the analysis of variance are not satisfied. *Biom Bull* **3**:22–38.

Cochran, W. G., 1947b, Recent developments in sampling theory in the United States. *Proc Inst Int Stat* **3A**:40–66.

Cochran, W. G., 1953a, *Sampling Techniques*. New York: John Wiley.

Cochran, W. G., 1953b, Statistical problems of the Kinsey Report. *J Am Stat Assoc* **48**: 673–716.

Cochran, W. G., 1967, Footnote by William G. Cochran. *Science* **156**:1460–62.

Cochran, W. G., 1976, Early development of techniques in comparative experimentation. In *On the History of Statistics and Probability*, D. B. Owen (ed.). New York: Marcel Dekker, pp. 3–25.

Cochran, W. G., 1979, Some reflections. *Biometrics* **35**:1–2.

Cochran, W. G., 1982, *Contributions to Statistics*. New York: John Wiley & Sons, p. 61.121.

Cochran, W. G., and Cox, G. M., 1946, Design of greenhouse experiments for statistical analysis. *Soil Sci* **62**:87–97.

Cochran, W. G., and Cox, G. M., 1950, *Experimental Designs*. New York: John Wiley.

Cochran, W. G., Mosteller, F., and Tukey, J. W., 1954, *Statistical Problems of the Kinsey Report*. Washington, D.C.: American Statistical Association.

Cole, P., 1980, Introduction. In *Statistical Methods in Cancer Research*, vol. 1, N. E. Breslow, N. E. Day (eds.), Lyon: International Agency for Research on Cancer, pp. 14–40.

Cole, P., and MacMahon, B., 1971, Attributable risk percent in case–control studies. *Br J Prev Soc Med* **25**:242–44.

Collins, R., Gray, R., Godwin, J., *et al.*, 1987, Avoidance of large biases and large random errors in the assessment of moderate treatment effects: The need for systematic overviews. *Stat Med* **6**:245–54.

Collins, R., Scrimgeour, A., Yusuf, S., *et al.*, 1988, Reduction in fatal pulmonary embolism and venous thrombosis by perioperative administration of subcutaneous heparin. Overview of results of randomized trials in general, orthopedic, and urologic surgery. *N Engl J Med* **318**:1162–73.

Collins, R., Peto, R., MacMahon, S., *et al.*, 1990, Blood pressure, stroke, and coronary heart disease. Part 2, Short-term reductions in blood pressure: Overview of randomised drug trials in their epidemiological context. *Lancet* **335**:827–38.

Colton, T., 1974, *Statistics in Medicine*. Boston: Little, Brown & Co., pp. 73–74.

Colton, T., 1981, Bill Cochran: His contributions to medicine and public health and some personal recollections. *Am Stat* **35**:167–70.

Committee for the Assessment of Biometric Aspects of Controlled Trials of Hypoglycemic Agents, 1975, Report. *JAMA* **231**:583–608.

Cook, E., 1925, *A Short Life of Florence Nightingale*, abridged by R. Nash. New York: Macmillan Co., p. 176.

Cope, A., 1958, Dr. William Farr, the medical statistician. In *Florence Nightingale and the Doctors*. London: Museum Press. Ch. 8.

Cornfield, J., 1951, A method of estimating comparative rates from clinical data. Applications to cancer of the lung, breast, and cervix. *J Natl Cancer Inst* **11**:1269–75.

Cornfield, J., 1976, Recent methodological contributions to clinical trials. *Am J Epidemiol* **104**:408–21.

Cox, D. R., 1958, The regression analysis of binary sequences. *J R Stat Soc B* **20**:215–42.

Cox, D. R., 1962, *Renewal Theory*. London: Methuen, pp. 1–24.

Cox, D. R., 1970, *The Analysis of Binary Data*. London: Methuen, pp. 87–90.

Cox, D. R., 1972, Regression models and life tables. *J. R. Stat Soc B* **34:**187–220.

Cox, D. R., and Oakes, D., 1984, *Analysis of Survival Data*. London: Chapman & Hall.

Craig, C. C., 1986, Early days in statistics at Michigan. *Stat Sci* **1:**292–93.

Cranberg, L., 1979, Do retrospective controls make clinical trials "inherently fallicious?" *Br Med J* **2:**1265–66.

Crombie, A. C., 1952, *Avicenna, Scientist and Philosopher*, G. M. Wickens (ed.). London: Luzac, p. 89. Reported in J. P. Bull, p. 221, 1959.

Crombie, A. C., 1961, *Augustine to Galileo*, vol. 1. London: Heinemann, p. 226.

Cunningham, A. S., 1988, Meta-analysis and methodology review: What's in a name? *J Pediatr* **113:**328–29.

Cutler, S. J., and Ederer, F., 1958, Maximum utilization of the life table method in analyzing survival. *J Chronic Dis* **8:**699–712.

Cuzick, J., Stewart, H., Peto, R., *et al.*, 1987, Overview of randomized trials comparing radical mastectomy without radiotherapy against simple mastectomy with radiotherapy in breast cancer. *Cancer Treat Rep* **71:**7–14.

Cuzick, J., Stewart, H. J., Peto, R., *et al.*, 1988, Overview of randomized trials of postoperative adjuvant radiotherapy in breast cancer. *Recent Results Cancer Res* **111:**108–29.

Dale, H., 1951, Measurement in medicine: Introduction. *Br Med Bull* **7:**261–63.

d'Alembert, J. L., 1761, *Réflexions sur le Calcul des Probabilités*. Opuscules II.

David, F. N., 1955, Dicing and gaming (a note on the history of probability). *Biometrika* **42:**1–15.

David, F. N., 1984, Discussion. In R. L. Plackett: Royal Statistical Society—the last 50 years, 1934–84. *J R Stat Soc A* **147**(2):140–50.

David, F. N., 1985, Karl Pearson. In *Encyclopedia of Statistical Sciences*, vol. 6, S. Kotz, N. L. Johnson (eds.). New York: John Wiley & Sons, pp. 653–55.

Deimel, R. F., 1953, Elasticity. In *Encyclopedia Americana*, vol. 10. New York: Americana Corp., pp. 48–54.

deMoivre, A., 1718, *The Doctrine of Chances, or a Method of Calculating the Probabilities of Events at Play*. London: Pearson.

DeVita, V. T., Jr., 1984, On special initiatives, critics, and the National Cancer Program. *Cancer Treat Rep* **68:**1–4.

DeVita, V. T., Jr., Serpick, A. A., and Carbone, P. P., 1970, Combination chemotherapy in the treatment of advanced Hodgkin's disease. *Ann Intern Med* **73:**881–95.

Dewey, D. R., 1889, The study of statistics. *Publ Am Econ Assoc* **4:**35–52.

Diamond, M., and Stone, M., 1981, Nightingale on Quetelet. *J R Stat Soc A* **144** (Part (1): 66–79.

Diehl, H. S., Baker, A. B., and Cowan, D. W., 1938, Cold vaccines: An evaluation based on a controlled study. *JAMA* **111:**1168–73.

Dodge, H. F., and Romig, H. G., 1929, A method of sampling inspection. *Bell Syst Tech J* **8:**613–31.

Doll, R., 1964, Retrospective and prospective studies. In *Medical Surveys and Clinical Trials*, 2nd ed., L. J. Witts (ed.). London: Oxford University Press, pp. 71–98.

Doll, R., 1979, Nutrition and cancer: A review. *Nutr Cancer* **1**(3):35–45.

Doll, R., 1992, Sir Austin Bradford Hill and the progress of medical science. *Br Med J* **305:**1521–26.

Doll, R., and Hill, A. B., 1950, Smoking and carcinoma of the lung. *Br Med J* **2**:739–48.

Doll, R., and Hill, A. B., 1952, A study of the aetiology of carcinoma of the lung. *Br Med J* **2**:1271–77.

Doll, R., and Hill, A. B., 1954, The mortality of doctors in relation to their smoking habits. A preliminary report. *Br Med J* **1**:1451–55.

Doll, R., and Peto, R., 1976, Mortality in relation to smoking: 20 years' observation on male British doctors. *Br Med J* **2**:1525–36.

Doll, R., and Peto, R., 1978, Cigarette smoking and bronchial carcinoma: Dose and time relationships among regular smokers and life-long non-smokers. *J Epidemiol Community Health* **32**:303–13.

Doll, R., Gray, R., Hafner, B., *et al.*, 1980, Mortality in relation to smoking: 22 years' observations on female British doctors. *Br Med J* **2**:967–71.

Drummond, J. C., and Wilbraham, A., 1940, *The Englishman's Food: A History of Five Centuries of English Diet*. London: Jonathan Cape.

Eastern Cooperative Group in Solid Tumor Chemotherapy, 1960, Appraisal of methods for the study of chemotherapy of cancer in man: Comparative therapeutic trial of nitrogen mustard and triethylene thiophosphoramide. *J Chronic Dis* **11**:7–33.

Eberbach, W. H., 1987, Individual cases and the scientific method—a conflict? Legal aspects of cancer clinical trials in the Federal Republic of Germany. *Recent Results Cancer Res* **111**:185–90.

Edgeworth, F. Y., 1881, *Mathematical Psychics*. London: Kegan Paul.

Edgeworth, F. Y., 1885, Methods of statistics. Jubilee volume of *Stat Soc*: 181–217.

Eisenberg, L., 1977, The social imperatives of medical research. *Science* **198**:1105–10.

Ellenberg, S. S., 1988, Meta-analysis: The quantitative approach to research review. *Semin Oncol* **15**:472–81.

Engberg, C. C., 1953, The statistical method. In *Encyclopedia Americana*, vol. 25. New York: Americana Corp., p. 531.

Eyler, J. M., 1971, *William Farr 1807–1883: An Intellectual Biography of a Social Pathologist*. Ph.D. thesis, University of Wisconsin.

Farber, S., Diamond, L. K., Mercer, R. D., *et al.*, 1948, Temporary remissions in acute leukemia in children prolonged by folic acid antagonist, 4-aminopteroylglutamic acid (aminopterin). *N Engl J Med* **238**:787–93.

Farr, W., 1837, Vital statistics, or the statistics of health, sickness, disease and death. In *Statistical Account of the British Empire*, McCulloch (ed.). London, pp. 567–601.

Farr, W., 1864, *English Life Table. Tables of Lifetimes, Annuities, and Premiums*. London: Longman.

Farr, W., 1885, *Vital Statistics*, a memorial volume of selections from the reports and writings of William Farr, N. A. Humphreys (ed.). London: Sanitary Institute, pp. vii–xxiv.

Feigl, P., and Zelen, M., 1965, Estimation of exponential survival probabilities with concomitant information. *Biometrics* **21**:826–38.

Feinstein, A. R., 1976, The persistent clinical failures and fallacies of the UGDP study. *Clin Pharmacol Ther* **19**:78–93.

Feinstein, A. R., 1984, Current problems and future challenges in randomized clinical trials. *Circulation* **70**:767–74.

Fisher, R. A., 1912, On an absolute criterion for fitting frequency curves. *Messeng Math* **41**:155–60.

Fisher, R. A., 1915, Frequency distribution of the values of the correlation coefficient in samples from an indefinitely large population. *Biometrika* **10**:507–21.

Fisher, R. A., 1918, The correlation to be expected between relatives on the supposition of Mendelian inheritance. *Trans R Soc Edinburgh* **52**:399–433.

Fisher, R. A., 1919, The genesis of twins. *Genetics* **4**:489–99.

Fisher, R. A., 1921, On the "probable error" of a coefficient of correlation deduced from a small sample. *Metron* **1**:3–32.

Fisher, R. A., 1922a, On the interpretation of chi-square from contingency tables, and the calculation of *P. J R Stat Soc* **85**:87–94.

Fisher, R. A., 1922b, On the dominance ratio. *Proc R Soc Edinburgh* **42**:321–41.

Fisher, R. A., 1924, The conditions under which chi-square measures the discrepancy between observation and hypothesis. *J R Stat Soc* **87**:442–50.

Fisher, R. A., 1925, 1928, 1930, 1932, 1934, 1936, 1938, 1941, 1944, 1946, 1950, 1954, 1958, 1970, *Statistical Methods for Research Workers*. Edinburgh: Oliver & Boyd.

Fisher, R. A., 1930, *The Genetical Theory of Natural Selection*. London: Oxford University Press. New York: Dover, 1958.

Fisher, R. A., 1934, Discussion. In J. Neyman: On the two different aspects of the representative method: The method of stratified sampling and the method of purposive selection, *J R Stat Soc* **97**:614–19.

Fisher, R. A., 1935, *The Design of Experiments*. Edinburgh: Oliver & Boyd, 8th ed. 1966. Reprinted New York: Hafner, pp. 6–7, 1971.

Fisher, R. A., 1939, "Student." *Ann Eugen* **9**:1–9.

Fisher, R. A., 1960, Scientific thought and the refinement of human reasoning. *J Oper Res Soc Jpn* **3**:1–10.

Fisher, R. A., 1971–74, *Collected Papers of R. A. Fisher*, 5 vols., J. H. Bennett (ed.). The University of Adelaide. [291 of Fisher's papers in chronologic order]

Fisher, R. A., and Ford, E. B., 1926, Variability of species. *Nature* **118**:515–16.

Fisher, R. A., and Ford, E. B., 1928, The variability of species in the *Lepidoptera*, with reference to abundance and sex. *Trans R Entomol Soc London* **76**:367–79.

Fisher, R. A., and Mackenzie, W. A., 1923, The manurial response of different potato varieties. *J Agric Sci* **13**:311–20.

Fitzpatrick, P. J., 1955, The early teaching of statistics in American colleges and universities. *Am Stat* **9**:12–18.

Fleming, T. R., 1992, Evaluating therapeutic interventions: Some issues and experiences. *Stat Sci* **7**:428–56.

Forrest, D. W., 1974, *Francis Galton: The Life and Work of a Victorian Genius*. New York: Taplinger, pp. 201–02.

Fost, N., 1979, Consent as a barrier to research. *N Engl J Med* **300**:1272–73.

Francis, T., Jr., Korns, R. F., Voight, R. B., et al., 1955, Evaluation of 1954 field trials of poliomyelitis vaccine, summary report. *Am J Public Health* **45**, No. 5

Frei, E., III, Holland, J. F., Schneiderman, M. A., et al., 1958, A comparative study of two regimens of combination chemotherapy in acute leukemia. *Blood* **13**:1126–48.

Frei, E., III, Freireich, E. J., Gehan, E., et al., 1961, Studies of sequential and combination antimetabolite therapy in acute leukemia: 6-mercaptopurine and methotrexate. *Blood* **18**:431–54.

Freireich, E. J., 1983, Methods for evaluating response to treatment in adult acute leukemia. *Blood Cells* **9**:5–20.

Freireich, E. J., and Gehan, E. A., 1979, The limitations of the randomized clinical trial. *Methods Cancer Res* **17**:277–310.

Freireich, E. J., Gehan, E. A., Frei, E., III, et al., 1963, The effect of 6-mercaptopurine on the duration of steroid-induced remissions in acute leukemia: A model for evaluation of other potentially useful therapy. *Blood* **21**:699–716.

Froggatt, P., and Nevin, N. C., 1971, The "law of ancestral heredity" and the Mendelian–ancestrian controversy in England 1889–1906. *J Med Genet* **8**:1–36.

Frost, W. H., 1965, Introduction to *Snow on Cholera*. New York: Hafner, p. xiv. [A reprint of two papers by Snow]

Galton, F., 1885, The application of a graphic method to fallible measures. Jubilee volume of *Stat Soc*: 262–65.

Galton, F., 1888, Co-relations and their measurement, chiefly from anthropometric data. *Proc R Soc* **45**:135–45.

Galton, F., 1889, *Natural Inheritance*. London: Macmillan, p. 62.

Galton, F., 1901, Biometry. *Biometrika* **1**:7–10.

Gart, J. J., 1972, Discussion of Cox (1972). *J R Stat Soc B* **34**:212, 219.

Gehan, E. A., 1959, Use of medical measurements to predict the course of disease. In *Conference on Experimental Clinical Cancer Chemotherapy*, B. H. Morrison, III (ed.). Bethesda: National Cancer Institute Monograph No. 3, pp. 51–58.

Gehan, E. A., 1961, The determination of the number of patients required in a preliminary and follow-up trial of a new chemotherapeutic agent. *J Chronic Dis* **13**:346–53.

Gehan, E. A., 1965, A generalized Wilcoxon test for comparing arbitrarily singly-censored samples. *Biometrika* **52**:203–23.

Gehan, E. A., 1969, Estimating survival functions from the life table. *J Chronic Dis* **21**:629–44.

Gehan, E. A., 1984, The evaluation of therapies: Historical control studies. *Stat Med* **3**:315–24.

Gehan, E. A., 1991, Statistics in cancer clinical trials. *Cancer Bulletin* (M. D. Anderson Cancer Center) **43**(3):268–74.

Gehan, E. A., and Freireich, E. J., 1974, Non-randomized controls in cancer clinical trials. *N Engl J Med* **290**:198–203.

Gehan, E. A., and Schneiderman, M. A., 1990, Historical and methodological developments in clinical trials at the National Cancer Institute. *Stat Med* **9**:871–80.

Gehan, E. A., Smith, T. L., Freireich, E. J., *et al.*, 1976, Prognostic factors in acute leukemia. *Semin Oncol* **3**:271–82.

Ghosh, B. K., 1988, Sequential analysis. In *Encyclopedia of Statistical Sciences*, vol. 8, S. Kotz, N. L. Johnson (eds.). New York: John Wiley & Sons, pp. 378–87.

Glass, G. V., 1976, Primary, secondary, and meta-analysis of research. *Educ Res* **6**:3–8.

Glover, J. W., 1926, Statistical teaching in American colleges and universities. *J Am Stat Assoc* **21**:419–24.

Goldenberg, I. S., McMahan, C. A., Escher, G. C., *et al.*, 1973, Secondary chemotherapy of advanced breast cancer. *Cancer* **31**:660–63.'

Gosset, W. S., 1970, *Letters from W. S. Gosset to R. A. Fisher 1915–1936*. Dublin: Arthur Guinness (private circulation).

Grattan-Guinness, I., 1978, Laplace. In *Dictionary of Scientific Biography*, vol. 15, suppl. 1, C. C. Gillespie (ed.). New York: Charles Scribner's Sons, p. 279.

Graunt, J., 1662, *Natural and Political Observations Made Upon the London Bills of Mortality*: With Reference to the Government, Religion, Trade, Growth, Ayr, Diseases, and the several Changes of the said City. London: Tho: Roycroft, for John Martin, James Allestry, and Tho: Dicas.

Green, S. B., 1982, Patient heterogeneity and the need for randomized clinical trials. *Controlled Clin Trials* **3:**189–98.

Greenspan, E. M., Fieber, M., Lesnick, G., *et al.*, 1963, Response of advanced breast carcinoma to the combination of the antimetabolite, methotrexate, and the alkylating agent, thio-TEPA. *J Mt Sinai Hosp* **30:**246–67.

Greenwald, P., 1988, Issues raised by the Women's Health Trial (editorial). *J Natl Cancer Inst* **80:**788–90.

Greenwood, M., 1924, Is the statistical method of any value in medical research? *Lancet* **2:**153–58.

Greenwood, M., 1941, Medical statistics from Graunt to Farr. *Biometrika* **32:**101–27.

Greenwood, M., 1942, Medical statistics from Graunt to Farr. *Biometrika* **32:**203–25.

Greenwood, M., 1943, Medical statistics from Graunt to Farr. *Biometrika* **33:**1–24.

Greenwood, M., Jr., and Yule, G. U., 1915, The statistics of anti-typhoid and anti-cholera inoculations and the interpretations of such statistics in general. *Proc R Soc Med* **8:** 113–94.

Gregg, N. M., 1941, Congenital cataract following German measles in the mother. *Trans Ophthalmol Soc Aust* **3:**35–46.

Gridgeman, N. T., 1971, Ronald Aylmer Fisher. In *Dictionary of Scientific Biography*, vol. 5. New York: Charles Scribner's Sons, pp. 7–11.

Guy, W. A., 1850, On the relative value of averages derived from different numbers of observations. *J Stat Soc* **13:**30–45.

Hald, A., 1990, *A History of Probability and Statistics and their Applications before 1750*. New York: John Wiley & Sons, p. 104.

Halley, E., 1693, An Estimate of the Degrees of Mortality of Mankind, drawn from curious Tables of the Births and Funerals at the City of Breslaw; with an Attempt to ascertain the Price of Annuities on Lives. *Philos Trans* **17:**596–610. (In a later collection printed in London: C. and R. Baldwin, New Bridge-Street, Blackfriars, 1809, this article is in *Philos Trans 1692–1693* **3:**483–91.

Halperin, M., DeMets, D. L., and Ware, J. H., 1990, Early methodological developments for clinical trials at the National Heart, Lung and Blood Institute. *Stat Med* **9:**881–92.

Hart, A., 1988, Standard deviation. In *Encyclopedia of Statistical Sciences*, vol. 8, S. Kotz, N. L. Johnson (eds.). New York: John Wiley & Sons, pp. 625–29.

Hawkins, F. B., 1829, *Elements of Medical Statistics*. London: Longman.

Haygarth, J., 1801, *Of the Imagination as a Cause and as a Cure of Disorders of the Body*. Bath: R. Crutwell, p. 3.

Haygarth, J., 1805, *A Clinical History of Diseases*. London: Cadell & Davies, p. 5.

Hellman, S., and Hellman, D. S., 1991, Of mice but not men: Problems of the randomized clinical trial. *N Engl J Med* **324:**1585–89.

Herbst, A. L., Ulfelder, H., and Poskanzer, D. C., 1971, Adenocarcinoma of the vagina: Association of maternal stilbestrol therapy with tumor appearance in young women. *N Engl J Med* **284:**878–81.

Hevly, B., 1990, A cultural tilt to science. *The Houston Chronicle*, October 29, p. 7B.

Hill, A. B., 1925, On the average longevity of physicians. *Br Med J* **1:**754–55.

Hill, A. B., 1929, An investigation of sickness in various industrial occupations. *J R Stat Soc* **92:**183–230.

Hill, A. B., 1936, The recent trend in England and Wales of mortality from phthisis of young adult ages. *J R Stat Soc* **99:**247–83.

Hill, A. B., 1937, *Principles of Medical Statistics*. London: Lancet Ltd. [12th ed. published shortly after he died with son I. D. Hill as coauthor]

Hill, A. B., 1950, Clinical trials of anti-histaminic drugs in the prevention and treatment of the common cold. *Br Med J* **2**:425–29.

Hill, A. B., 1951a, The doctor's day and pay. *J R Stat Soc A* **114**:1–34.

Hill, A. B., 1951b, The clinical trial. *Br Med Bull* **7**:278–82.

Hill, A. B., 1952, The clinical trial. *N Engl J Med* **247**:113–19.

Hill, A. B., 1953, Observation and experiment. *N Engl J Med* **248**:995–1001.

Hill, A. B., 1955, Snow—An appreciation. *Proc R Soc Med* **48**:1008–12.

Hill, A. B., 1957, Smoking and cancer of the lung (letter). *Lancet* **2**:1289.

Hill, A. B., 1963, Medical ethics and controlled trials. *Br Med J* **1**:1043–49.

Hill, A. B., 1965, The environment and disease: Association or causation? *Proc R Soc Med* **58**:295–300.

Hill, A. B., 1966, Reflections on the controlled trial. *Ann Rheum Dis* **25**:107–13.

Hill, A. B., 1968, The life of Sir Leonard Erskine Hill FRS (1866–1952). *Proc R Soc Med* **61**:307–16.

Hill, A. B., 1971, Diseases of treatment. *Public Health* **85**:197–202.

Hill, A. B., 1982, Is bran useful in diverticular disease? (letter). *Br Med J* **284**:46.

Hill, A. B., 1983, A pilot in the first world war. *Br Med J* **287**:1947–49.

Hill, A. B., 1987, Clinical trials and the acceptance of uncertainty (letter). *Br Med J* **294**:1419.

Hill, A. B., 1990, Memories of the British streptomycin trial in tuberculosis. *Controlled Clin Trials* **11**:77–79.

Hill, A. B., and Doll, R., 1956, Lung cancer and tobacco. *Br Med J* **1**:1160–63.

Hill, A. B., and Doll, R., 1960, Deaths from lung cancer (letter). *Lancet* **1**:1292.

Hill, A. B., and Faning, E. L., 1948, Studies in incidence of cancer in factories handling inorganic compounds of arsenic: Mortality experience in the factory. *Br J Ind Med* **5**:1–6.

Hill, A. B., and Galloway, T. M., 1949, Maternal rubella and congenital defects. *Lancet* **1**:299–301.

Hill, A. B., and Knowelden, J., 1950, Inoculation and poliomyelitis: A statistical investigation in England and Wales in 1949. *Br Med J* **2**:1–6.

Hill, A. B., and Martin, W. J., 1949, Poliomyelitis and social environment. *Br Med J* **2**:357–58.

Hill, A. B., Hatswell, J. M., and Topley, W. W. C., 1940, The inheritance of resistance, demonstrated by the development of a strain of mice resistant to experimental inoculation with a bacterial endotoxin. *J Hyg* **40**:538–47.

Hill, A. B., Doll, R., and Galloway, T. M., 1958, Virus diseases in pregnancy and congenital defects. *Br J Prev Soc Med* **12**:1–7.

Hill, G. B., 1983, Controlled clinical trials—The emergence of a paradigm. *Clin Invest Med* **6**:25–32.

Hill, I. D., 1982, Austin Bradford Hill: Ancestry and early life. *Stat Med* **1**:297–300.

Hill, I. D., 1984, Royal Statistical Society: The first 100 years, 1834–1934. *J R Stat Soc A* **147**(2):130–39.

Hill, I. D., 1988, Royal Statistical Society. In *Encyclopedia of Statistical Sciences*, vol. 8, S. Kotz, N. L. Johnson (eds.). New York: John Wiley & Sons, pp. 206–07.

Himsworth, Sir Harold, 1982, Bradford Hill and statistics in medicine. *Stat Med* **1**:301–03.

Hinkley, D. V., 1980, R. A. Fisher: Some introductory remarks. In *R. A. Fisher: An Appreciation*, S. E. Fienberg, D. V. Hinkley (eds.). Berlin: Springer-Verlag, pp. 1–5.

Historical exhibits, 1940, *J Am Stat Assoc* **35:**298, 303–04.

Hoeffding, W., 1978, Harold Hotelling. In *International Encyclopedia of Statistics*, vol 1, W. H. Kruskal, J. M. Tanur (eds.). New York: The Free Press, pp. 439–41.

Hotelling, H., 1927, Differential equations subject to error, and population estimates. *J Am Stat Assoc* **22:**283–314.

Hotelling, H., 1931a, The generalization of Student's ratio. *Ann Math Stat* **2:**360–78.

Hotelling, H., 1931b, Frequency distributions. In *Encyclopedia of the Social Sciences*, vol. 6. New York: Macmillan Co., pp. 484–89.

Hotelling, H., 1933, Analysis of a complex of statistical variables into principal components. *J Educ Psychol* **24:**417–41, 498–520.

Hotelling, H., 1935, The most predictable criterion. *J Educ Psychol* **26:**139–42.

Hotelling, H., 1936, Relations between two sets of variates. *Biometrika* **28:**321–77.

Hotelling, H., 1940, The teaching of statistics. *Ann Math Stat* **11:**457–70. Reprinted in *Stat Sci* **3:**63–71, 1988.

Hotelling, H., 1941, Experimental determination of the maximum of a function. *Ann Math Stat* **12:**20–45.

Hotelling, H., 1942a, Problems of prediction. *Am J Sociol* **48:**61–76.

Hotelling, H., 1942b, Foreword to *Tables of Probability Functions*, vol. II. Washington, D.C.: National Bureau of Standards, U. S. Government Printing Office.

Hotelling, H., 1947, Multivariate quality control, illustrated by the air testing of sample bombsights. In *Selected Techniques of Statistical Analysis*, C. Eisenhart, M. W. Hastay, W. A. Wallis (eds.). New York: McGraw–Hill, Ch. 3.

Hotelling, H., 1949, The place of statistics in the university. In *Proceedings of the Berkeley Symposium on Mathematical Statistics and Probability*, J. Neyman (ed.). Berkeley: University of California Press, pp. 21–40. Reprinted in *Stat Sci* **3:**72–83, 1988.

Hotelling, H., 1951, A generalized T test and measure of multivariate dispersion. In *Proceedings of the Second Berkeley Symposium on Mathematical Statistics and Probability*, J. Neyman (ed.). Berkeley: University of California Press, pp. 23–42.

Hotelling, H., and Hotelling, F., 1931. Causes of birth rate fluctuations. *J Am Stat Assoc* **26:**135–49.

Hotelling, H., and Hotelling, F., 1932, A new analysis of duration of pregnancy data. *Am J Obstet Gynecol* **23:**643–57.

Hoyle, E., 1754, *An Essay towards Making the Doctrine of Chances Easy to Those who Understand Vulgar Arithmetic Only*. London: Jolliff.

Hoyle, E., 1770, *Mr. Hoyle's Games of Whist, Quadrille, Piquet, Chess, and Backgammon, complete. In Which are Contained the Method of Playing and Betting at these Games, upon Equal or Advantageous Terms. Including the Laws of Several Games*, 15th ed. London: Osborne.

Huguley, C. M., Jr., Durant, J. R., Moores, R. R., *et al.*, 1975, A comparison of nitrogen mustard, vincristine, procarbazine, and prednisone (MOPP) vs. nitrogen mustard in advanced Hodgkin's disease. *Cancer* **36:**1227–40.

Hunter, J., 1794, *A Treatise on the Blood, Inflammation and Gun-Shot Wounds*. London: G. Nicol, pp. 531–38.

Huygens, C., 1657, *De Ratiociniis in Ludo Aleae*. Netherlands: van Schooten.

Ingraham, H. S., 1958, Statistics and medical knowledge. *Am J Public Health* **48:**1449–59.

Jenner, E., 1798, *An Inquiry into the Causes and Effects of the Variolae Vaccinae, a Disease Discovered in some of the Western Counties of England, particularly Gloucestershire, and known by the name of The Cow Pox*. London: S. Low.

Kaplan, E. L., and Meier, P., 1958, Nonparametric estimation from incomplete observations. *J Am Stat Assoc* **53**:457–81.

Kargon, R., 1963, John Graunt, Francis Bacon, and the Royal Society: The reception of statistics. *J Hist Med Allied Sci* **18**:337–48.

Keating, M. J., Smith, T. L., Gehan, E. A., *et al.*, 1980, Factors related to length of complete remission in adult acute leukemia. *Cancer* **45**:2017–29.

Keefer, C. S., Blake, F. G., Marshall, E. K., Jr., *et al.*, 1943, Penicillin in the treatment of infections: A report of 500 cases. *JAMA* **122**:1712–24.

Kendall, M. G., 1956, The beginnings of a probability calculus. *Biometrika* **43**:1–14.

Kendall, M. G., 1961, Daniel Bernoulli on maximum likelihood. *Biometrika* **48**:1–2.

Kendall, M. G., 1963, Ronald Aylmer Fisher, 1890–1962. *Biometrika* **50**:1–15.

Kendall, M. G., 1970, Francis Ysidro Edgeworth, 1845–1926. In *Studies in the History of Statistics and Probability*, E. S. Pearson, M. G. Kendall (eds.). New York: Hafner, pp. 257–63.

Kendall, M. G., 1972, The history and future of statistics. In *Statistical Papers in Honor of George W. Snedecor*. Ames: Iowa State University Press, pp. 193–210.

King, L. S., 1964, The so-called scientific method: Some historical considerations. *Surgery* **56**:450–58.

Kinsey, A. C., Pomeroy, W. B., and Martin, C. E., 1948, *Sexual Behavior in the Human Male*. Philadelphia: W. B. Saunders.

Kruskal, W. H., and Wallis, W. A., 1952, Use of ranks in one-criterion variance analysis. *J Am Stat Assoc* **47**:583–621.

Lachin, J. M., 1988, Statistical properties of randomization in clinical trials. *Controlled Clin Trials* **9**:289–311.

Lane-Claypon, J. E., 1926, A further report on cancer of the breast, with special reference to its associated antecedent conditions. *Reports on Public Health and Medical Subjects*, No. 32. London: Her Majesty's Stationery Office, pp. 1–189.

Laplace, P.-S., 1812, *Théorie Analytique des Probabilités*. Paris: Ve. Courcier.

Lasagna, L., 1955, The controlled clinical trial: Theory and practice. *J Chronic Dis* **1**:353–58.

Lehmann, E. L., 1990, Jerzy Neyman. In *Dictionary of Scientific Biography* **18**(Suppl. 2): 669–75.

Lehmann, E. L., 1993, The Fisher, Neyman–Pearson theories of testing hypotheses: One theory or two? *J Am Stat Assoc* **88**:1242–49.

Levene, H., 1974, Howard Hotelling. *Am Stat* **28**:71–73.

Levine, R. J., 1991, Comment on R. M. Royall: Ethics and statistics in randomized clinical trials. *Stat Sci* **6**:71–74.

Lew, E. A., 1985, Actuarial contributions to life table analysis. *Natl Cancer Inst Monogr* **67**:29–36.

Lexis, W., 1877, *Zur Theorie der Massenerscheinungen in der menschlichen Gesellschaft*. Wagner, Feiburg im Breisgau.

Lilienfeld, A. M., and Lilienfeld, D. E., 1980, The 1979 Heath Clark Lectures, "The epidemiologic fabric." I. Weaving the threads. *Int J Epidemiol* **9**:199–206.

Lind, J., 1753, *A Treatise of the Scurvy*. Edinburgh: Sands, Murray & Cochran. Reprinted by C. P. Stewart and D. Guthrie (eds.), Edinburgh University Press, pp. 145–58, 1953.

Lindley, F., 1991, Comment on R. M. Royall: Ethics and statistics in randomized clinical trials. *Stat Sci* **6**:74–77.

Lister, J., 1870, On the effects of the antiseptic system of treatment upon the salubrity of a surgical hospital. *Lancet* **1**:4–6, 40–42.

Locke, J., 1677, Letter to Dr. Maplelott, as quoted in B. Stookey and J. Ransohoff: *Trigeminal Neuralgia: Its History and Treatment*. Springfield, Ill: Charles C Thomas, pp. 8–10, 1959.

Lord, C. F. J., dictated 1889, The sanitary experiences of Charles F. J. Lord, M.R.C.S. In *Jottings: Some Experiences with Reflections Derived Through Life and Work in Hampstead from 1827 to 1877*, pamphlet vol. 3807. Washington, D.C.: Library of the Surgeon-General, pp. 36–37.

Louis, P. C. A., 1825, *Researches on Phthisis: Anatomical, Pathological and Therapeutical*. London: C. and J. Adlard, translated for the Sydenham Society, pp. xi–xxx, 1843.

Louis, P. C. A., 1834, *Essay on Clinical Instruction*, translated by P. Martin. London: S. Highley, pp. 26–28.

Louis, P. C. A., 1835, *Recherches sur les effets de la saignée dans quelques maladies inflammatoires: et sur l'action de l'emetique et des vesicatoires dans la pneumonie*. Paris: J. B. Baillière. Translated by C. G. Putnam, Boston: Hillary Gray, p. 1, 1836.

Lush, J. L., 1972, Early statistics at Iowa State University. In *Statistical Papers in Honor of George W. Snedecor*, T. A. Bancroft (ed.). Ames: Iowa State University Press, pp. 211–26.

MacMahon, S., Collins, R., Peto, R., *et al.*, 1988, Effects of prophylactic lidocaine in suspected acute myocardial infarction. An overview of results from the randomized, controlled trials. *JAMA* **260:**1910–16.

MacMahon, S., Peto, R., Cutler, J., *et al.*, 1990, Blood pressure, stroke, and coronary heart disease. Part 1. Prolonged differences in blood pressure: Prospective observational studies corrected for the regression dilution bias. *Lancet* **335:**765–74.

Mainland, D., 1954, The rise of experimental statistics and the problems of a medical statistician. *Yale J Biol Med* **27:**1–10.

Malgaigne, J. F., 1840–1841, *Oeuvres Complètes d'Ambroïse Paré*, vol. 2. Paris, p. 127. Reported in Mettler, p. 845, 1947.

Mann, H. B., and Whitney, D. R., 1947, On a test of whether one of two random variables is stochastically larger than the other. *Ann Math Stat* **18:**50–60.

Mann, J., 1964, *Louis Pasteur: Founder of Bacteriology*. New York: Charles Scribner's Sons.

Mantel, N., 1966, Evaluation of survival data and two new rank order statistics arising in its consideration. *Cancer Chemother Rep* **50:**163–70.

Mantel, N., and Haenszel, W., 1959, Statistical aspects of the analysis of data from retrospective studies of disease. *J Natl Cancer Inst* **22:**719–48.

Marshall, E. K., Jr., and Merrell, M., 1949, Clinical therapeutic trial of a new drug. *Bull Johns Hopkins Hosp* **85:**221–30.

Mason, R. L., McKenzie, J. D., Jr., and Ruberg, S. J., 1990, A brief history of the American Statistical Association, 1839–1989. *Am Stat* **44:**68–73.

Mather, C., 1722, *An Account of the Method and Success of Inoculating the Small-Pox in Boston in New England*. London: Peele.

May, L. A., 1977, *Withering on the Foxglove and other Classics in Pharmacology*. Oceanside: Dabor, pp. v–xxi.

McCance, R. A., 1951, Practice of experimental medicine. *Proc R Soc Med* **44:**189–94.

Medical Research Council, 1931, Clinical trials of new remedies (annotations). *Lancet* **2:**304.

Medical Research Council, 1948, Streptomycin treatment of pulmonary tuberculosis. *Br Med J* **2:**769–82.

Medical Research Council, 1951, The prevention of whooping cough by vaccination. *Br Med J* **1**:1463–71.

Meier, P., 1984, William G. Cochran and public health. In *W. G. Cochran's Impact on Statistics*, P. S. R. S. Rao, J. Sedransk (eds.). New York: John Wiley & Sons, pp. 73–81.

Meinert, C. L., 1986, *Clinical Trials: Design, Conduct, and Analysis*, C. L. Meinert (ed.). London: Oxford University Press, p. 5.

Mettler, C. C., 1947, *History of Medicine*, F. A. Mettler (ed.). Philadelphia: Blakiston, p. 192.

Mood, A. M., 1990, Miscellaneous reminiscences. *Stat Sci* **5**:35–43.

Moore, D. S., 1988, Comment. *Stat Sci* **3**:84–87.

Morton's Medical Bibliography, 1991, 5th ed., J. M. Norman (ed.). London: Cambridge University Press, p. 264.

Newell, D. J., 1984, Present position and potential developments: Some personal views—medical statistics. *J R Stat Soc A* **147**(2):186–97.

Neyman, J., 1934, On the two different aspects of the representative method: The method of stratified sampling and the method of purposive selection. *J R Stat Soc* **97**:558–625.

Neyman, J., 1937, Outline of a theory of statistical estimation based on the classical theory of probability. *Philos Trans R Soc London Ser A* **236**:333–80.

Neyman, J., 1938, *Lectures and Conferences on Mathematical Statistics and Probability*. Washington, D.C.: U. S. Department of Agriculture. 2nd ed., 1952.

Neyman, J., 1961, Silver jubilee of my dispute with Fisher. *J Oper Res Soc Jpn* **3**:145–54.

Neyman, J., 1974, *The Heritage of Copernicus: Theories 'Pleasing to the Mind.'* Cambridge, Mass: MIT Press.

Neyman, J., 1976, The emergence of mathematical statistics: A historical sketch with particular reference to the United States. In *On the History of Statistics and Probability*, D. B. Owen (ed.). New York: Marcel Dekker, pp. 149–93.

Neyman, J., and Pearson, E. S., 1928, On the use and interpretation of certain test criteria for purposes of statistical inference. *Biometrika* **20-A**:175–240, 263–94.

Neyman, J., and Pearson, E. S., 1933, On the problem of the most efficient tests of statistical hypotheses. *Philos Trans R Soc Ser A* **231**:289–337.

Nightingale, F., 1858, *Notes on Matters Affecting the Health, Efficiency, and Hospital Administration of the British Army*. Privately printed for Miss Nightingale, Harrison & Sons.

Nightingale, F., 1860, *Hospital Statistics*. Programme of the Fourth Session of the International Statistical Congress, London, July. London: Eyre & Spottiswoode.

Nightingale, F., 1864, *Observations on the Evidence Contained in the Stational Reports Submitted to the Royal Commission on the Sanitary State of the Army in India*. Reprinted from the Report of the Royal Commission, Edward Stanford.

Noether, G. E., 1989, The teaching of statistics in the USA: The early years. In *Proc Am Stat Assoc Sesquicentennial Invited Papers Session* pp. 279–85.

O'Fallon, W. M., 1988, A historical perspective of statistics. *Mayo Clin Proc* **63**:952–54.

Olschewski, M., Verres, R., Scheurlen, H., *et al.*, 1988, Evaluation of psychosocial aspects in a breast preservation trial. *Recent Results Cancer Res* **111**:258–69.

Pack, G. T., and Ariel, I. M., 1960, *Tumors of the Breast, Chest and Esophagus*, G. T. Pack, I. M. Ariel (eds.). New York: Harper & Row (Hoeber).

Paracelsus, 1951, *Selected Writings*, J. Jacobi (ed.), translated by N. Guterman. London: Routledge & Kegan Paul, p. 126.

Patulin Clinical Trials Committee (of the Medical Research Council), 1944, Clinical trial of Patulin in the common cold. *Lancet* **2**:373–75.

Pearson, E. S., 1934, Discussion. In J. Neyman: On the two different aspects of the representative method: The method of stratified sampling and the method of purposive selection, *J R Stat Soc* **97**:610–11.

Pearson, E. S., 1937, Karl Pearson: An appreciation of some aspects of his life and work, part II. *Biometrika* **29**:161–248.

Pearson, E. S., 1965, Studies in the history of probability and statistics. XIV. Some incidents in the early history of biometry and statistics, 1890–94. *Biometrika* **52**:3–18.

Pearson, E. S., 1970, The Neyman–Pearson story: 1926–34. In *Studies in the History of Statistics and Probability*, E. S. Pearson, M. G. Kendall (eds.). New York: Hafner, pp. 455–77.

Pearson, K., 1894, Contributions to the mathematical theory of evolution. *Philos Trans A* **185**:71–110.

Pearson, K., 1900, On the criterion that a given system of deviation from the probable in the case of a correlated system of variables is such that it can be reasonably supposed to have arisen from random sampling. *Philos Mag* Ser 5 **50**:157–72.

Pearson, K., 1930, *Life, Letters and Labours of Francis Galton*, vol. 3A. London: Cambridge University Press, p. 241.

Pearson, K., 1978, *The History of Statistics in the 17th and 18th Centuries*, E. S. Pearson (ed.). New York: Macmillan Co., p. 365.

Pearson, K., and Lee, A., 1903, On the laws of inheritance in man. *Biometrika* **2**:357–462.

Peters, W. S., 1987, *Counting for Something: Statistical Principles and Personalities*. Berlin: Springer-Verlag, p. 44.

Peto, J., and Easton, D., 1989, Cancer treatment trials—Past failures, current progress and future prospects. *Cancer Surv* **8**:511–33.

Peto, J., Eden, O. B., Lilleyman, J., *et al.*, 1986, Improvement in treatment for children with acute lymphoblastic leukaemia. The Medical Research Council UKALL Trials, 1972–84. *Lancet* **1**:408–11.

Petty, W., 1662, *Treatise on Taxes and Contributions*. London: Printed for N. Brooke, at the Angel in Cornhill.

Petty, W., 1755, *Several Essays in Political Arithmetick: with Memoirs of the Author's Life*. London: Routledge Thoemmes Press, 1992.

Petty, W., 1755, *The Petty Papers*, 2 vols., Marquis of Lansdowne (ed.). London: Constable, 1927.

Pocock, S. J., 1976, The combination of randomized and historical controls in clinical trials. *J Chronic Dis* **29**:175–88.

Pocock, S. J., 1977, Group sequential methods in the design and analysis of clinical trials. *Biometrika* **64**:191–99.

Pollock, H. M., 1953, Statistics. In *Encyclopedia Americana*, vol. 25. New York: Americana Corp., p. 536b.

Prentice, R. L., 1991, Aspects of the science of cancer prevention trials: Lessons from the conduct and planning of clinical trials of a low-fat diet intervention among women. *Prev Med* **20**:147–57.

Prentice, R. L., Self, S. G., and Mason, M. W., 1986, Design options for sampling within a cohort. In *Modern Statistical Methods in Chronic Disease Epidemiology*, S. H. Moolgavkar, R. L. Prentice (eds.). New York: John Wiley & Sons, pp. 50–62.

Quetelet, A., 1835, *Sur l'homme et le développement de ses facultés, ou Essai de physique sociale*. Paris; Bachelier, p. 12.

Quetelet, A., 1842, *A Treatise on Man and the Development of His Faculties*. Edinburgh: Chambers, p. 6. Translation of Quetelet, 1835.

Rao, P. S. R. S., 1984, Cochran's contributions to variance components models for combining estimates. In *W. G. Cochran's Impact on Statistics*, P. S. R. S. Rao, J. Sedransk (eds.). New York: John Wiley & Sons, pp. 203–21.

Read, C. B., 1983, William Sealy Gosset ("Student"). In *Encyclopedia of Statistical Sciences*, vol. 3, S. Kotz, N. L. Johnson (eds.). New York: John Wiley & Sons, pp. 461–63.

Rehn, L., 1895, Blasengeschwülste bei Fuchsin-Arbeitern. *Arch Klin Chir* 50:588–600.

Reid, C., 1982, *Neyman—From Life*. Berlin: Springer-Verlag, p. 79.

Rheumatic Fever Working Party of the Medical Research Council of Great Britain and the Subcommittee of Principal Investigators of the American Council on Rheumatic Fever and Congenital Heart Disease, 1960, The evolution of rheumatic heart disease in children: Five-year report of a cooperative clinical trial of ACTH, cortisone, and aspirin. *Circulation* 22:503–15.

Richardson, B. W., 1887, John Snow, M.D.: A representative of medical science and art of the Victorian era. *Aesculapiad* 4:274–300. Reprinted in *Snow on Cholera*, New York: Hafner, pp. xxv–xlviii, 1965.

Rietz, H. L., 1927, *Mathematical Statistics*. New York: Mathematical Association of America, Carus Mathematical Monographs.

Rosner, F., 1987, The ethics of randomized clinical trials. *Am J Med* 82:283–90.

Sacks, H. S., Berrier, J., Reitman, D., et al., 1992, Meta-analysis of randomized controlled trials: An update of the quality and methodology. In *Medical Uses of Statistics*, 2nd ed., J. C. Bailar III, F. Mosteller (eds.). Boston: NEJM Books, pp. 427–42.

Schmidt, B. C., 1977, Five years into the National Cancer Program: Retrospective perspectives—the National Cancer Act of 1971. *J Natl Cancer Inst* 59:687–92.

Schneiderman, M., 1982, A personal reminiscence. *Stat Med* 1:307–08.

Scott, E., 1985, Jerzy Neyman. In *Encyclopedia of Statistical Sciences*, vol. 6, S. Kotz, N. A. Johnson (eds.). New York: John Wiley & Sons, pp. 215–23.

Sessoms, S. M., 1960, Review of the Cancer Chemotherapy National Service Center Program: Development and organization. *Cancer Chemother Rep* 7:25–64.

Sheynin, O. B., 1977, D. Bernoulli's work on probability. In *Studies in the History of Statistics and Probability*, vol. 2, M. Kendall, R. L. Plackett (eds.). New York: Macmillan Co., pp. 105–32.

Shorter, E., 1987, *The Health Century*. New York: Doubleday, pp. 179–211.

Shryock, R. H., 1979, *The Development of Modern Medicine*. New York: Knopf, pp. 135–69.

Simon, R., and Wittes, R. E., 1985, Methodologic guidelines for reports of clinical trials. *Cancer Treat Rep* 69:1– 3.

Smalley, R. V., Murphy, S., Huguley, C. M., Jr., et al., 1976, Combination versus sequential five-drug chemotherapy in metastatic carcinoma of the breast. *Cancer Res* 36:3911–16.

Smith, T. L., Gehan, E. A., Keating, M. J., et al., 1982, Prediction of remission in adult acute leukemia: Development and testing of predictive models. *Cancer* 50:466–72.

Smith, W. L., 1978, Harold Hotelling 1895–1973. *Ann Stat* 6:1173–83.

Snedecor, G. W., 1937, *Statistical Methods Applied to Experiments in Agriculture and Biology*, Ames: Iowa State College Press.

Snedecor, G. W., and Cochran, W. G., 1967, *Statistical Methods*, 6th ed. Ames: Iowa State University Press.

Snow, J., 1855, *On the Mode of Communication of Cholera*. London: Churchill, pp. 1–139. Reprinted in *Snow on Cholera*. New York: Hafner, pp. 1–139, 1965.

Soper, H. E., Young, A. W., Cave, B. H., *et al.*, 1917, On the distribution of the correlation coefficient in small samples. Appendix II to the papers of "Student" and R. A. Fisher. A cooperative study. *Biometrika* **11**:328–413.

Sprat, T., 1722, *History of the Royal Society.* London, p. 67.

Steiner, W. R., 1940, Dr. Pierre-Charles-Alexander Louis, a distinguished Parisian teacher of American medical students. *Ann Med Hist* **2**:451–60.

Stigler, S. M., 1986, *The History of Statistics: The Measurement of Uncertainty before 1900.* Cambridge, Mass.: Belknap of Harvard University Press, p. 17.

Stinnett, S., and Collaborators, 1990, Women in statistics. *Am Stat* **44**:74–80.

"Student," 1908, The probable error of a mean. *Biometrika* **6**:1–25.

"Student," 1936, Co-operation in large-scale experiments. *J R Stat Soc* (Suppl) **3**:115–36.

"Student," 1937, Comparison between balanced and random arrangements of field plots. *Biometrika* **29**:363–79.

Sutherland, I., 1963, John Graunt: A tercentenary tribute. *J R Stat Soc A* **126**:537–56.

Sutow, W. W., Gehan, E. A., Dyment, P. G., *et al.*, 1978, Multidrug adjuvant chemotherapy for osteosarcoma: Interim report of the Southwest Oncology Group studies. *Cancer Treat Rep* **62**:265–69.

Taton, R., 1963, *The Beginnings of Modern Science*, vol. 2, translated by A. J. Pomerans. New York: Basic Books, pp. 547–48.

Taylor, K. M., and Kelner, M., 1987, Informed consent: The physicians' perspective. *Soc Sci Med* **24**:135–43.

Thomson, A. L., 1973, *Half a Century of Medical Research, vol. 1: Origin and Policy of the Medical Research Council (UK).* London: Her Majesty's Stationery Office, p. 136.

Underwood, E. A., 1951, The history of the quantitative approach in medicine. *Br Med Bull* **7**:265–74.

University Working Group Diabetes Program, 1970, A study of the effects of hypoglycemic agents on vascular complications in patients with adult-onset diabetes. II. Mortality. *Diabetes* **19**:785–830.

Vallery-Radot, R., 1923, *The Life of Pasteur*, translated by R. L. Devonshire. Garden City: Garden City Publishing, pp. 311–22.

van der Linden, W., 1980, Pitfalls in randomized surgical trials. *Surgery* **87**:258–62.

van Helmont, J. B., 1662, *Oriatrike or Physik Refined*, translated by J. Chandler. London: Lodowick Loyd. Quoted in Debus, A. G., 1968, *The Chemical Dream of the Renaissance.* Cambridge: Heffer, p. 72. Also quoted in Armitage, 1982.

Verstraete, M., 1979, Introduction to *The Challenge of Clinical Trials in Thrombosis*, M. Verstraete, J. Vermylen, H. Roberts (eds.). Stuttgart: Schattauer Verlag, pp. xi–xiii.

Villeneuve, A., 1990, Ethics and clinical drug trials. *Encephale* **16**:281–82.

Wald, A., 1943, Statistical Research Group Report No. 75. New York: Columbia University.

Wald, A., 1947, *Sequential Analysis.* New York: John Wiley & Sons, pp. 1–4.

Wald, A., 1950, *Statistical Decision Functions.* New York: John Wiley & Sons.

Wald, A., and Wolfowitz, J., 1940, On a test whether two samples are from the same population. *Ann Math Stat* **11**:147–62.

Walker, F. A., 1890, The study of statistics in colleges and technical schools. *Technol Q* **3**:1–8.

Walker, F. A., 1897, Remarks of President Walker at Washington. *Publications of the ASA* **5**:180–87. Reprinted in *Discussions in Economics and Statistics*, vol. II. New York: Augustus M. Kelley Publishers, *Reprints of Economic Classics*, 1971.

Walker, H. L., 1929, *Studies in the History of Statistical Method.* Baltimore: Williams & Wilkins, pp. 172–74.

Walker, H. L., 1958, The contributions of Karl Pearson. *J Am Stat Assoc* **53**:11–22.

Wallace, H. A., and Snedecor, G. W., 1925, *Correlation and Machine Calculations.* Ames: Publications of Iowa State College of Agriculture and Mechanics, vol. 23, No. 35.

Watson, G. S., 1982, William Gemmell Cochran 1909–1980. *Ann Stat* **10**:1–10.

Weiss, L., 1988, Abraham Wald. In *Encyclopedia of Statistical Sciences*, vol. 9, S. Kotz, N. L. Johnson (eds.). New York: John Wiley & Sons, pp. 514–17.

Weldon, W. F. R., 1890, The variations occurring in certain *Decapod Crustacea.* I: *Crangon vulgaris.* Proc R Soc **47**:445–53.

Weldon, W. F. R., 1892, Certain correlated variations in *Crangon vulgaris. Proc R Soc* **51**:2–21.

Weldon, W. F. R., 1906, Inheritance in animals and plants. In *Lectures on the Method of Science*, T. B. Strong (ed.). London: Oxford University Press (Clarendon), pp. 81–109.

Westergaard, H., 1932, *Contributions to the History of Statistics.* New York: Agathon Press, pp. 100–12, 1968.

Whitehead, J. R., 1983, *The Design and Analysis of Sequential Clinical Trials.* Chichester: Ellis Horwood, p. 21.

Wilcoxon, F., 1945, Individual comparisons by ranking methods. *Biom Bull* **1**:80–83.

Wilcoxon, F., 1947, Probability tables for individual comparisons by ranking methods. *Biometrics* **3**:119–22.

Wilcoxon, F., and Wilcox, R. A., 1947, 1949, *Some Rapid Approximate Statistical Procedures.* Pearl River, NY: Stamford Research Laboratories, 1964.

Williams, C. J. B., 1884, *Memoirs of Life and Work of Charles J. B. Williams.* London, p. 43.

Withering, W., 1785, *An Account of the Foxglove, and Some of its Medical Uses: with Practical Remarks on Dropsy and Other Diseases.* Birmingham: C. G. J. & J. Robinson, p. vi.

Woodham-Smith, C., 1950, *Florence Nightingale.* New York: McGraw–Hill, p. 180.

Wright, C. D., 1888, The study of statistics in colleges. *Publ Am Econ Assoc* **3**:5–28.

Wynder, E. L., Cornfield, J., Schroff, P. D., *et al.*, 1954, A study of environmental factors in carcinoma of the cervix. *Am J Obstet Gynecol* **68**:1016–52.

Yates, F., 1982, Obituary: William Gemmell Cochran, 1909–1980. *J R Stat Soc* **145**:521–23.

Young, A., 1771, *A Course of Experimental Agriculture.* Dublin: J. Exshaw *et al.*

Yule, G. U., 1911, *An Introduction to the Theory of Statistics*, London: Griffin, pp. 82, 202, 14th ed. 1950.

Yule, G. U., 1922, An application of the chi-square method of association and contingency tables, with experimental illustrations. *J R Stat Soc* **85**:95–104.

Yusuf, S., Collins, R., MacMahon, S., *et al.*, 1988, Effect of intravenous nitrates on mortality in acute myocardial infarction: An overview of the randomised trials. *Lancet* **1**: 1088–92.

Zelen, M., 1979, A new design for randomized clinical trials. *N Engl J Med* **300**:1242–45.

Zelen, M., Gehan, E., and Glidewell, O., 1980, Biostatistics. In *Cancer Research: Impact of the Cooperative Groups*, B. Hoogstraten (ed.). Paris: Masson, pp. 291–312.

Zidek, J. V., 1988, Comment. *Stat Sci* **3**:87–90.

Zubrod, C. G., 1979, Historic milestones in curative chemotherapy. *Semin Oncol* **6**:490–505.

Name Index

Subject Index